The Surf Girl Guide To
Surf Fitness

An inspirational guide to FITNESS & WELL-BEING for girls who surf

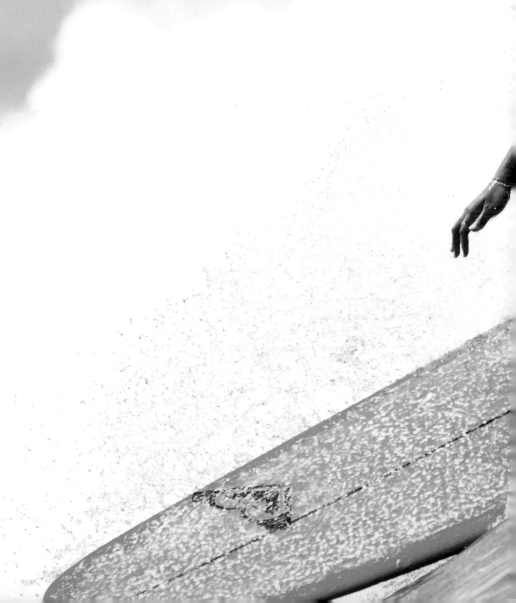

FITTER • FASTER • STRONGER •

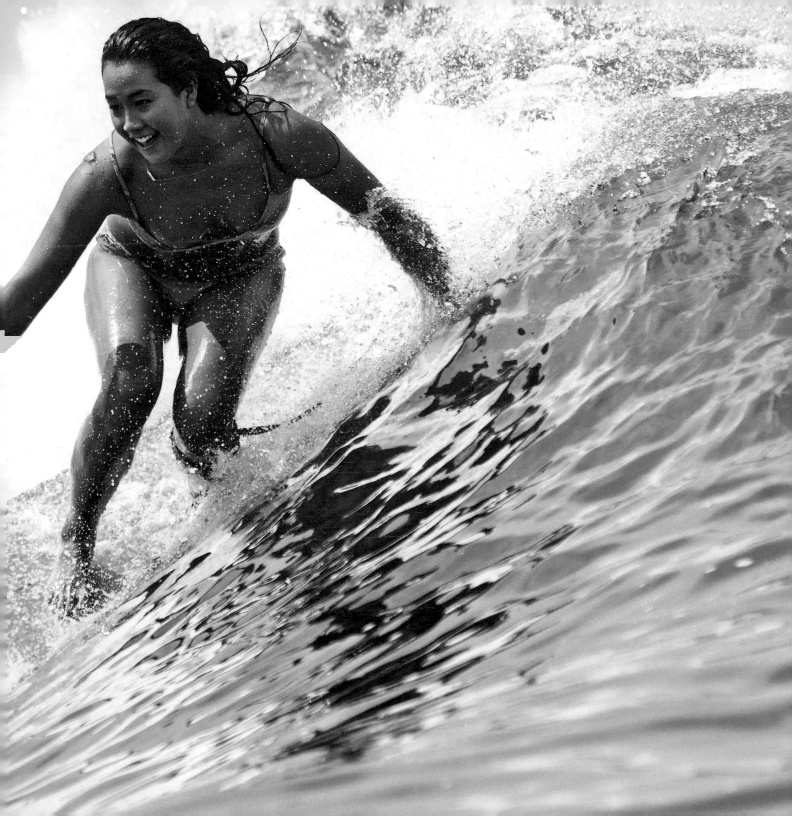

staff

The Surf Girl Guide To Surf Fitness
ISBN 978-0-9567893-7-2

Copyright ©2015 Orca Publications Limited.
All rights reserved. No part of this book may be reproduced in any form without written permission from the publisher.

Printed and bound: Great Wall Printing, Hong Kong
Published by Orca Publications Limited, Berry Road Studios, Berry Road, Newquay, TR7 1AT, United Kingdom.
www.orcasurf.co.uk • +44 (0) 1637 878074

surfgirl   **orca**publications

This book wouldn't have been possible without the help and support of the following people:

Editor Louise Searle
Editorial Consultant Lee Stanbury
Sub Editor Hayley Spurway
Senior Designer David Alcock
Design Assistant Chelsea Holter
Photography Roger Sharp, Mike Searle, Abbi Hughes, Simon Williams, Samantha Bass, Mike Morgan, Katie Watson, Morgan Maassen, Mikala Wilbow, Fellipe Ditadi
Contributors Lee Stanbury, Aimee Stapleford, Natalie Fox, Natalie Frankson, Katie Watson, Samantha Bass, Hayley Shaw McGuinness
Consultants Steve England, Chris Power
Proofreader Alex Hapgood
Fitness Model Jessica Davis

Cover: Stephanie Gilmore. Photo: Richard Kotch. Back cover photo: Zacher/ROXY.

IN ASSOCIATION WITH

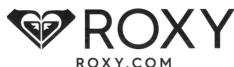

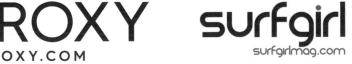

4

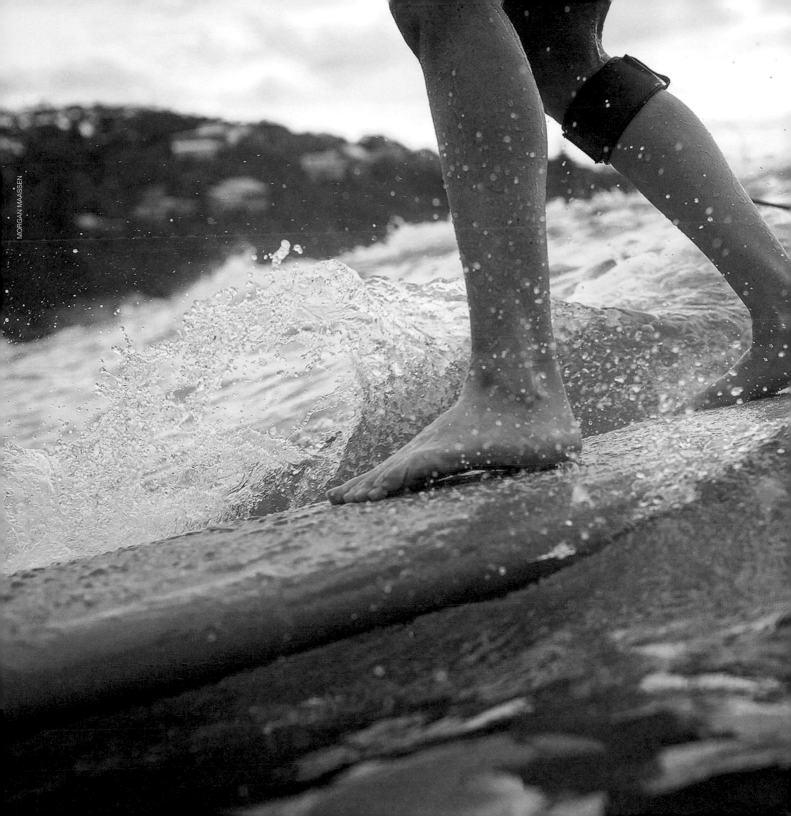

contents

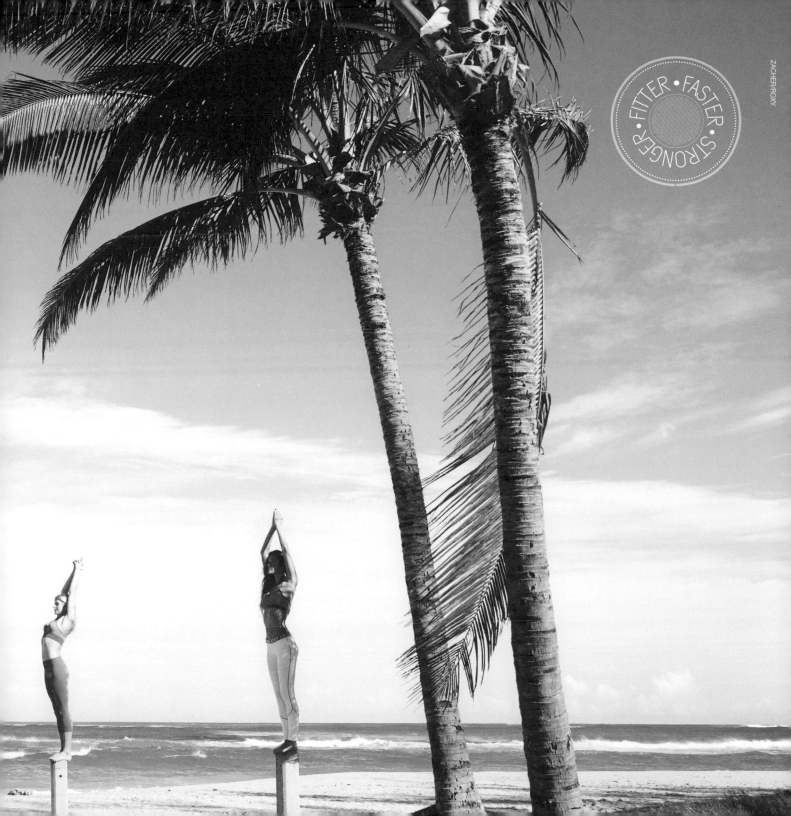

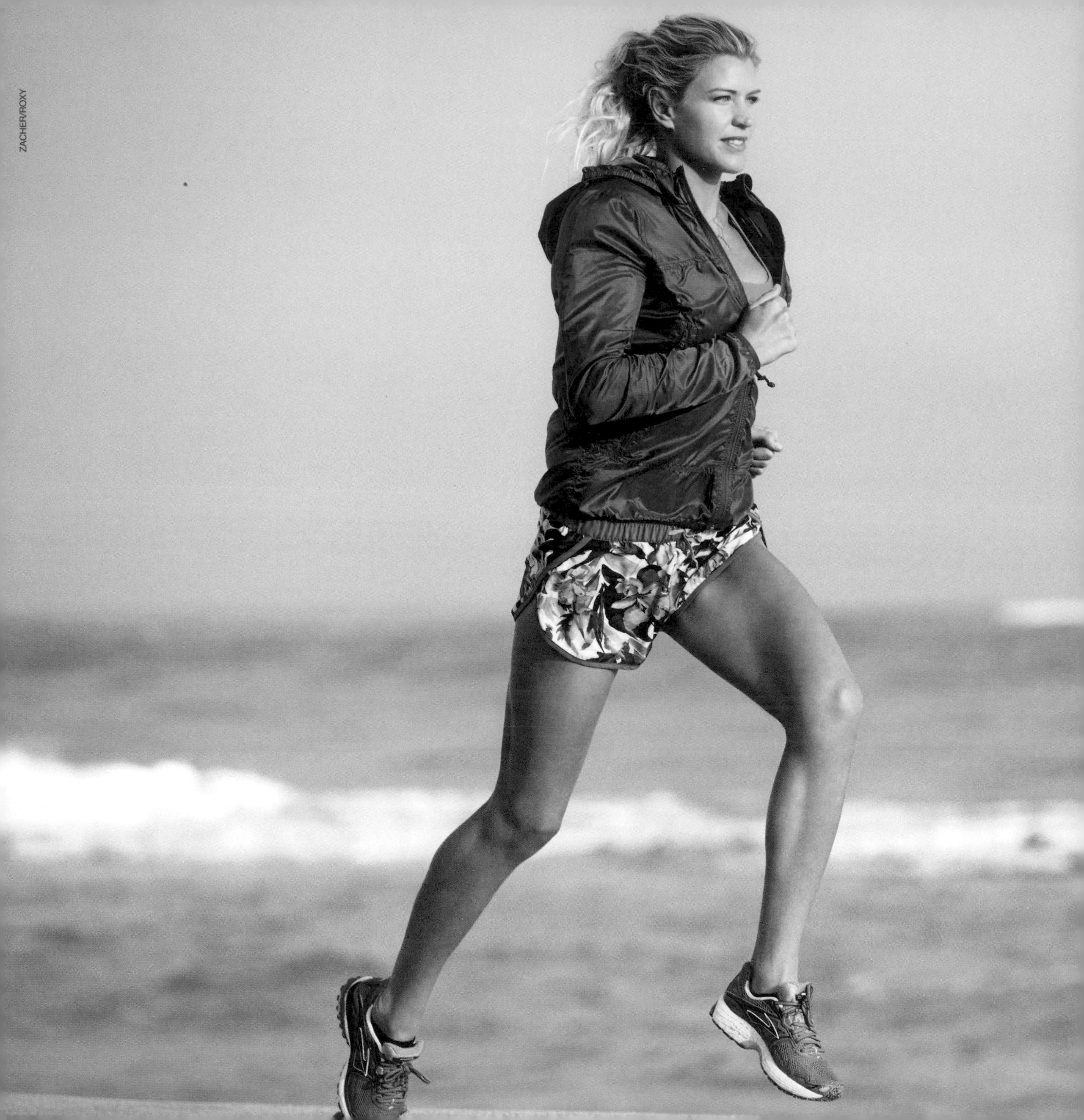
ZACHER/ROXY

foreword

When I was about 10 years old I used to go to 'surf team training' twice a week. I absolutely hated running up and down the dunes while there were waves breaking in the distance. But I remember the older boys telling me that training would make me a better surfer, and they also said I needed to run off all the candy I'd eaten – because I've always had a sweet tooth!

Fast forward 10 years, and when I finished school I was able to travel the world, call myself a professional athlete and get sponsored by Roxy. One of the key things I learnt about training was that putting a few hours a week into making myself physically and mentally stronger benefitted me and my surfing. Whether you want to become more confident in the water or make a dash for a world title, training is vital. I always try and get myself into gear, make an effort to workout, and I'm always improving and learning.

So, my advice? Go and get sweaty, then jump in the water to wash it all away!

Rosy Hodge

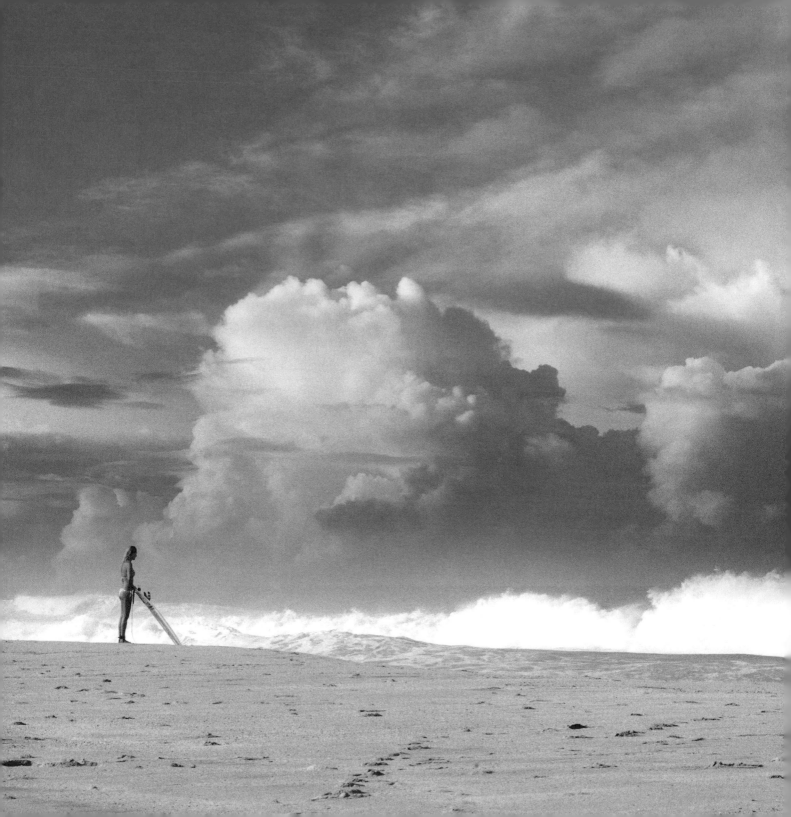

CHALLENGE YOURSELF. TOMORROW STARTS TODAY.

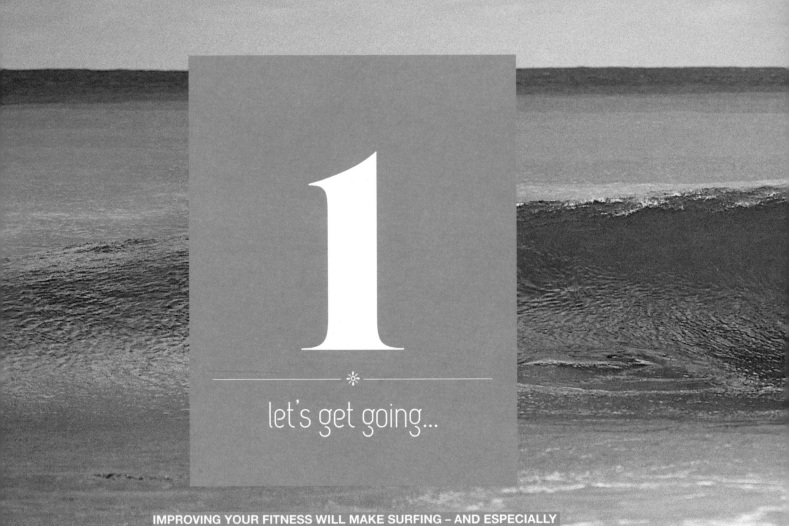

1

*

let's get going...

IMPROVING YOUR FITNESS WILL MAKE SURFING – AND ESPECIALLY
LEARNING TO SURF – MUCH MORE ENJOYABLE, HERE'S HOW.

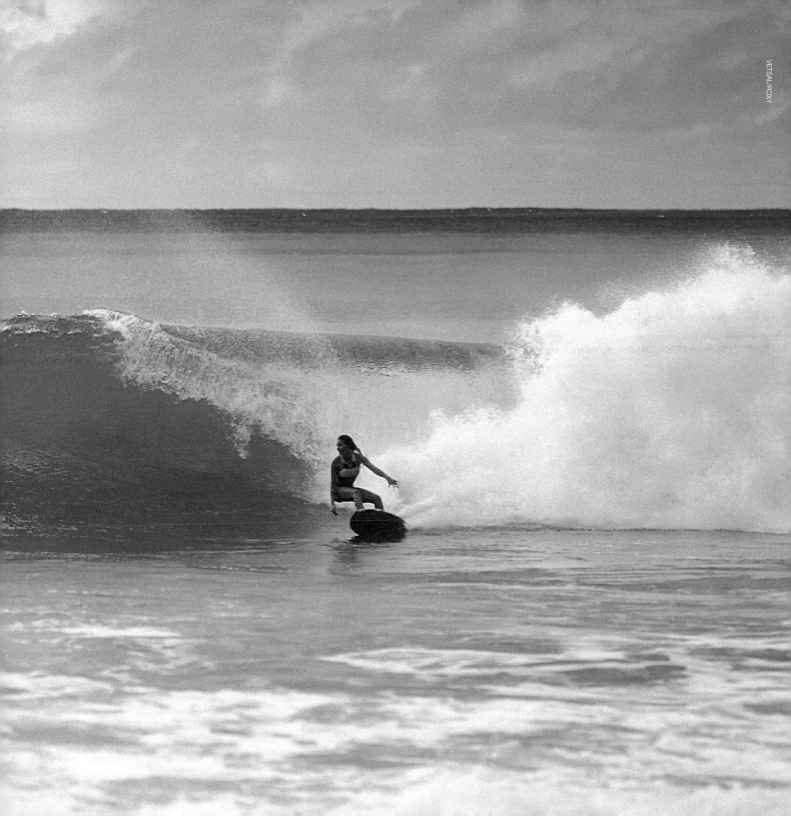

why training benefits your surfing

Surfing is a demanding sport – what with all that paddling, all those wipeouts and the strength you need to pull off manoeuvres when you're up and riding a wave. Even getting in and out of your wetsuit can be exhausting if you're not fit.

Improving your fitness will make surfing – and especially learning to surf – much more enjoyable. It will increase your stamina and power to catch more waves, enable you to spend more time in the water, improve basic surfing manoeuvres and help you to deal with the challenging conditions the ocean can throw at you.

When you're training, try to focus on the muscle groups specific to surfing movements – this is called sports specific training.

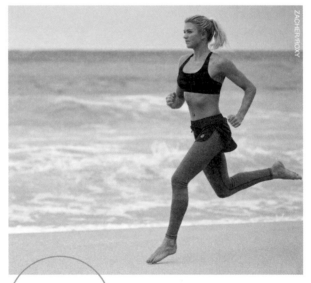

ZACHER/ROXY

Benefits of exercise

» IMPROVED CARDIO FITNESS

» FASTER RECOVERY TIMES

» IMPROVED PERFORMANCE

» CONFIDENCE BOOST

» STRONGER SURFING MOVEMENTS

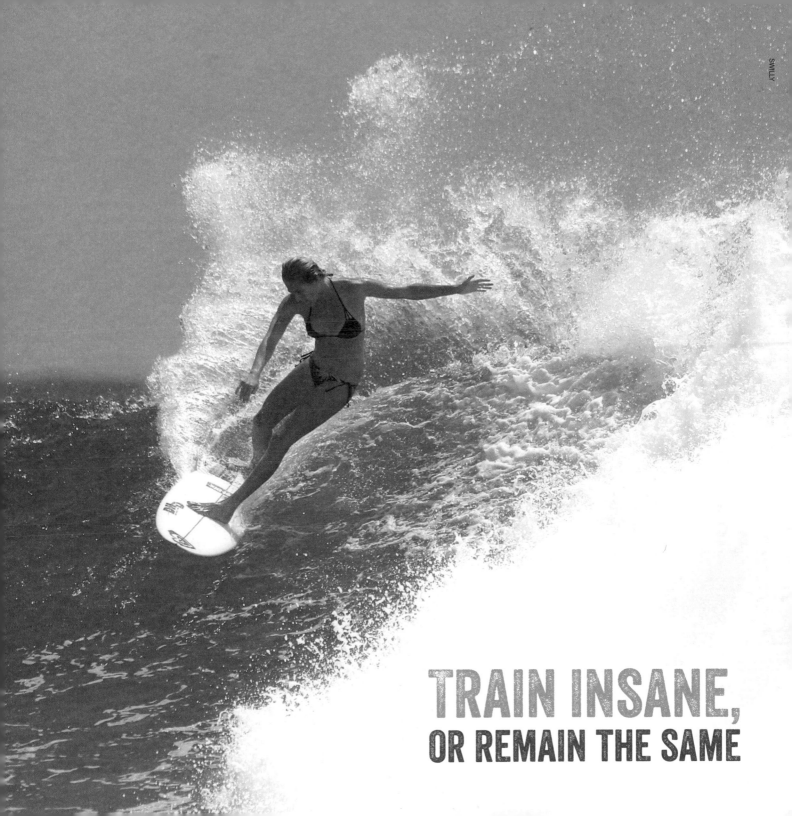

SWILLY

TRAIN INSANE,
OR REMAIN THE SAME

So what does it all mean?

Terminology

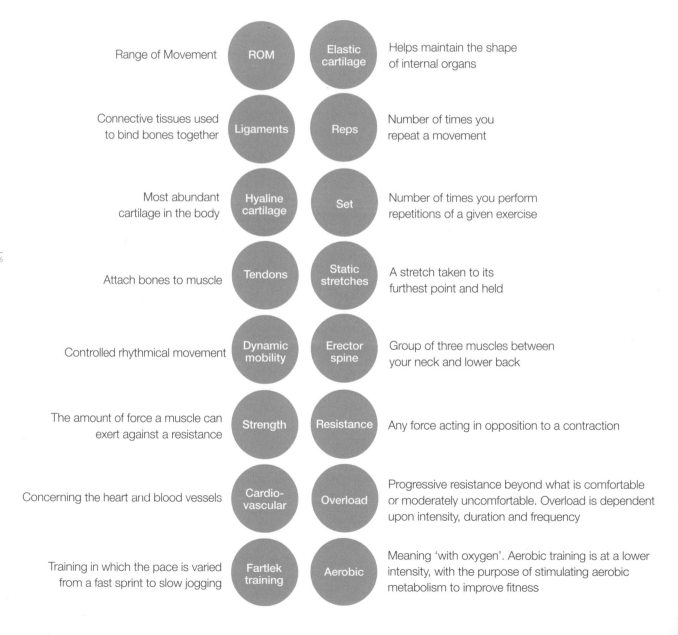

Range of Movement — **ROM**

Elastic cartilage — Helps maintain the shape of internal organs

Connective tissues used to bind bones together — **Ligaments**

Reps — Number of times you repeat a movement

Most abundant cartilage in the body — **Hyaline cartilage**

Set — Number of times you perform repetitions of a given exercise

Attach bones to muscle — **Tendons**

Static stretches — A stretch taken to its furthest point and held

Controlled rhythmical movement — **Dynamic mobility**

Erector spine — Group of three muscles between your neck and lower back

The amount of force a muscle can exert against a resistance — **Strength**

Resistance — Any force acting in opposition to a contraction

Concerning the heart and blood vessels — **Cardio-vascular**

Overload — Progressive resistance beyond what is comfortable or moderately uncomfortable. Overload is dependent upon intensity, duration and frequency

Training in which the pace is varied from a fast sprint to slow jogging — **Fartlek training**

Aerobic — Meaning 'with oxygen'. Aerobic training is at a lower intensity, with the purpose of stimulating aerobic metabolism to improve fitness

the warm up

BEFORE SURFING OR STARTING ANY EXERCISE SESSION, IT'S ESSENTIAL TO WARM UP. WHY?

1. Warming up makes tissues more pliable and ready to exercise, and therefore makes injuries less likely.
2. The body works more efficiently when warm. It reaches a steady state of energy production and your performance will improve.

A decent warm up should be continuous and rhythmical, should last between 4-8 minutes, and should include a gentle exercise for the whole body – such as light jogging – to gradually increase the heart rate, breathing and blood supply to the muscles. Additional light mobility exercises such as arm swings and leg swings can warm up your muscles and help to prepare you for your first wave.

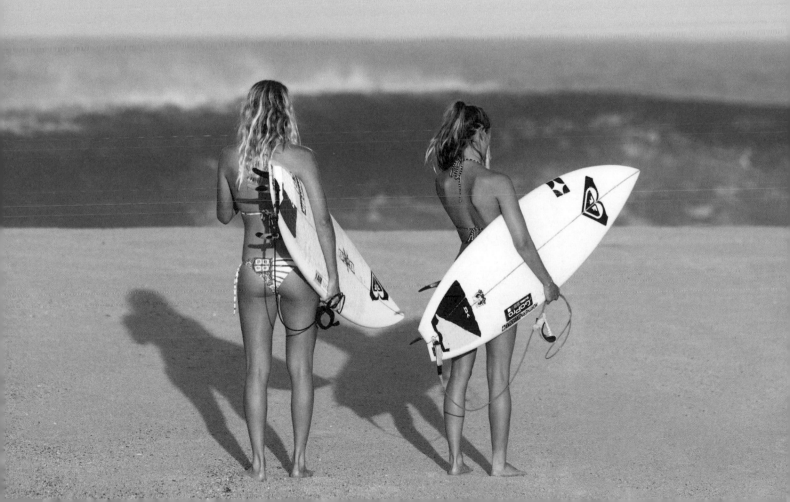

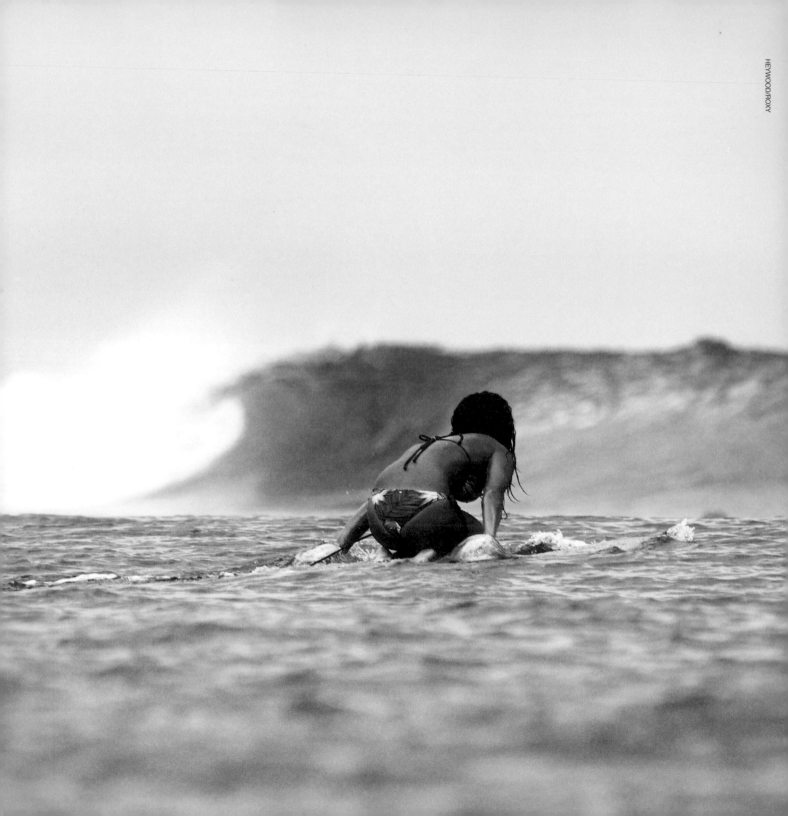

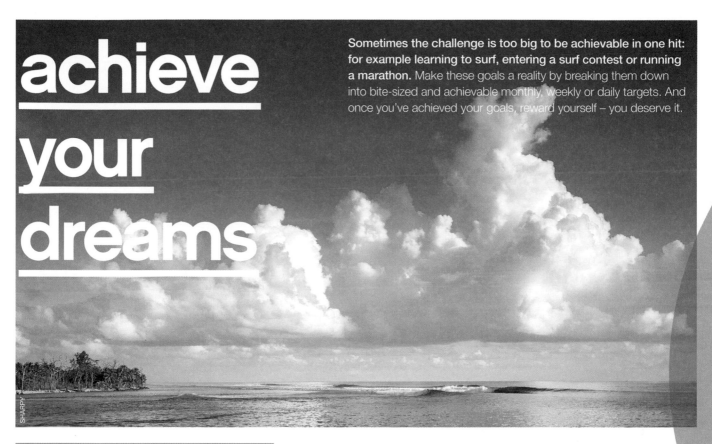

achieve your dreams

Sometimes the challenge is too big to be achievable in one hit: for example learning to surf, entering a surf contest or running a marathon. Make these goals a reality by breaking them down into bite-sized and achievable monthly, weekly or daily targets. And once you've achieved your goals, reward yourself – you deserve it.

SHARPY

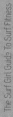

PRIORITISE YOUR STEPPING STONES TO SUCCESS

Not enough time to achieve what you really want? Then make a list of your goals and write down daily or weekly steps to reach them. Cut down on other activities that aren't bringing you benefits – organise your time and you'll find you have more time to achieve your goals.

"Great things are done by a series of small things brought together."

VINCENT VAN GOGH

MAKE A LIST LIKE THIS

GOAL	TIMING	REWARD

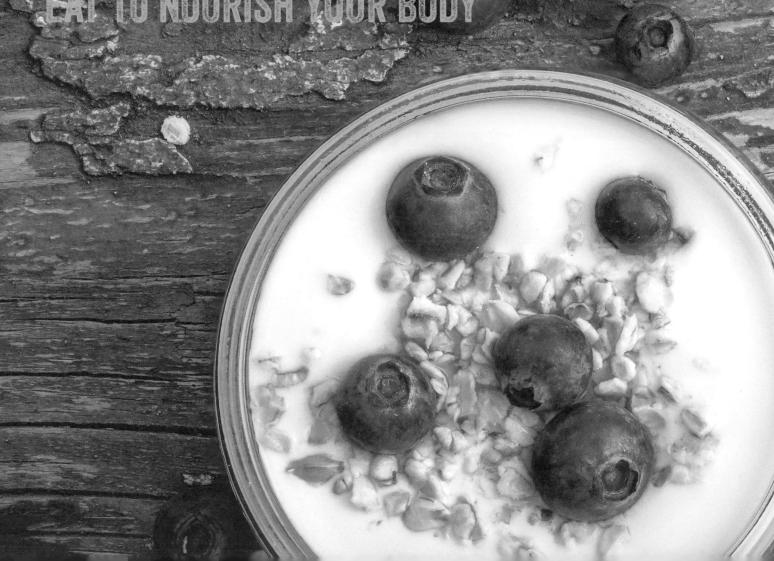

BAN THE MUNCHIES...
EAT TO NOURISH YOUR BODY

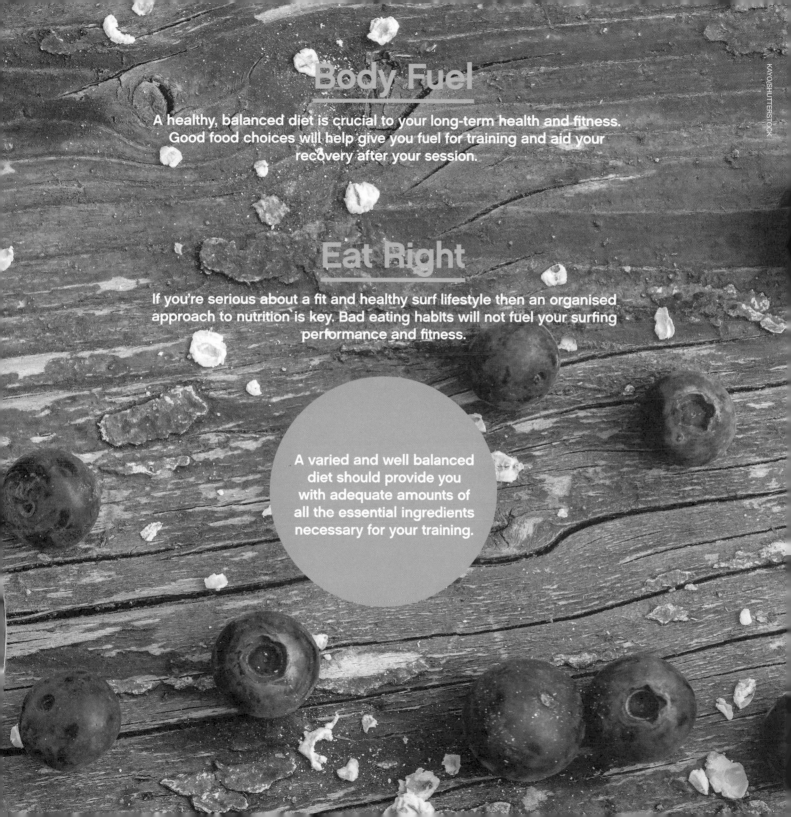

Body Fuel

A healthy, balanced diet is crucial to your long-term health and fitness. Good food choices will help give you fuel for training and aid your recovery after your session.

Eat Right

If you're serious about a fit and healthy surf lifestyle then an organised approach to nutrition is key. Bad eating habits will not fuel your surfing performance and fitness.

A varied and well balanced diet should provide you with adequate amounts of all the essential ingredients necessary for your training.

The Good Food List

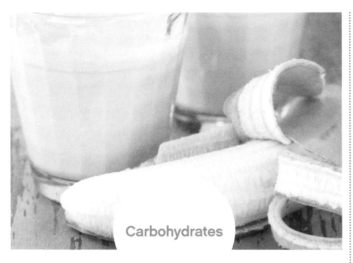

Carbohydrates

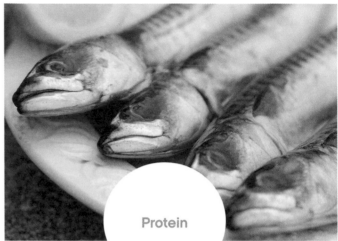

Protein

Carbohydrates are the key ingredients for creating energy. During intensive activity periods the focus should be on eating carbs so that your energy tank is full and ready for take-off. They need to be regularly topped up, as our stores of carbs are small. It's the most important energy fuel and crucial for sustaining training and recovery.

Good sources of carbohydrates:

Sweet potatoes	Dried apricots
Rice	Cashew nuts
Cous cous	Low-fat yoghurt
Boiled and new potatoes	Apple juice
Pumpkin	Orange juice
Baked beans	
Wholegrain and rye bread	
Muesli	
Oatmeal	
Whole-wheat pasta	
Lentils	
Brown rice	
Bananas	
Apples	

Protein plays an important part in building and repairing muscle, so it is vital that a varied diet provides enough protein. A portion of protein is recommended within 30 minutes of exercise. Animal sources are richer than vegetable sources (so a larger quantity of non-animal sources needs to be consumed). Eggs are a good choice because they provide a good balance of protein and fat, as are fish like salmon or haddock and low-fat dairy foods. Protein-rich foods break down more slowly, which means you stay fuller for longer.

Good sources of protein:

Chicken and turkey	Yoghurt
Pork	Cheese
Fish	Cereal
Soya beans	Broccoli
Tofu	Tuna
Lentils	Bananas
Kidney beans	
Baked beans	
Pistachio nuts	
Eggs	
Milk	

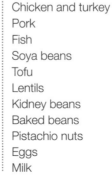

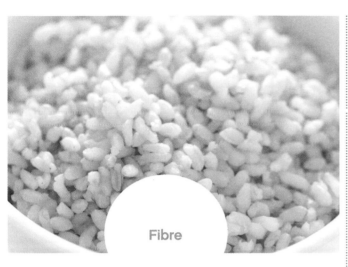

Fibre

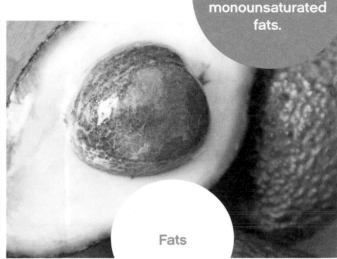

Fats

If you're surfing regularly and training hard you will need a good amount of fibre in your diet. High fibre foods are a great source of vitamins and minerals, and also help prevent bowel problems. High fibre foods also fill you up for longer, can help keep weight down, and also help prevent heart disease by lowering cholesterol.

Good sources of fibre:

Porridge
Lentils
Beans
Oats
Chickpeas
Walnuts

Jacket potato
Wheat bran
Wholegrain cereals
Brown rice
Fruit and vegetables

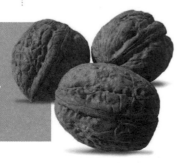

Walnuts are a nutrient-dense food: 100 grams of walnuts contain 15.2 grams of protein, 65.2 grams of fat, and 6.7 grams of dietary fibre.

Avocados contain about 10% monounsaturated fats.

Fats play a highly important role in your fitness nutrition. Fats and oils are made of fatty acids and serve as a rich source of energy for the body. Your body breaks down fats and uses them to store energy, insulate your body and transport vitamins through the bloodstream. It is true to say, however, that some fats are better than others!

• Monounsaturated fats are found mainly in vegetable oils, like olive oil and some peanut oils.

• Polyunsaturated fats are found mainly in vegetable oils like safflower, sunflower, corn and flaxseed. They are also the main fats found in seafood.

• Saturated fats are mainly found in animal sources like meats, poultry, milk and cheese.

• Trans-fatty acids can be formed when vegetable oils are processed into margarine or shortening. Sources of these trans fats include snack foods and baked goods made with partially hydrogenated vegetable oil or vegetable shortening.

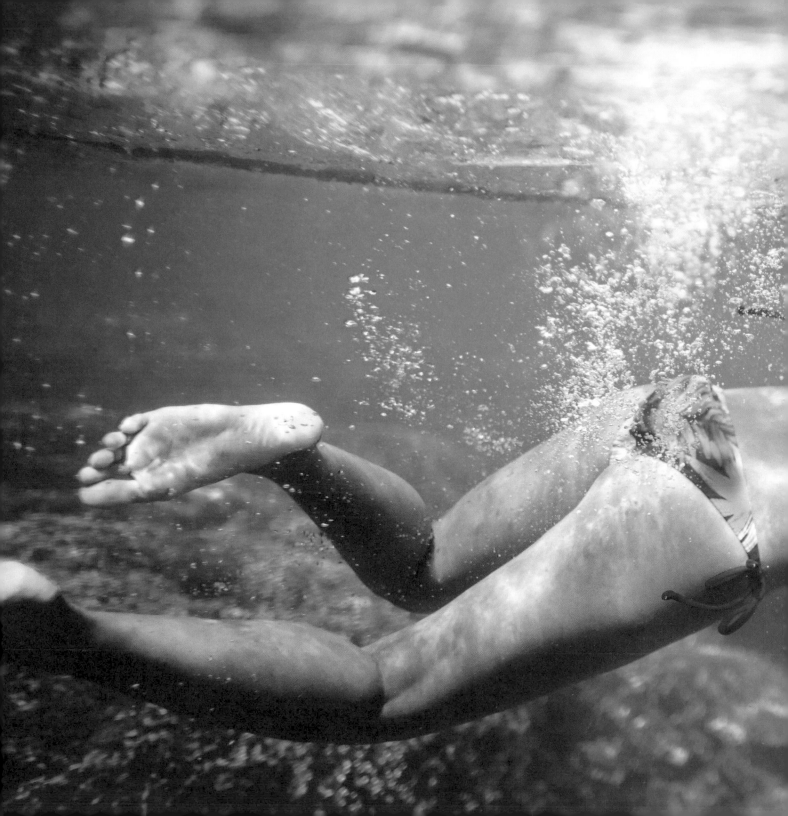

REWARD YOURSELF

WHEN YOU'VE ACHIEVED YOUR GOALS. AN INCENTIVE WILL HELP KEEP YOU MOTIVATED ON YOUR ROAD TO SUCCESS.

A Balanced Diet

Eat a wide variety of foods to ensure all your micronutrient requirements are met. You should get used to combining protein, fat and carbs in each meal or snack.
You need starchy carbs for breakfast and lunch to fuel activity, but for your evening meal the carbs should be replaced by vegetables. You don't have to eat enormous meals to achieve this balance, in fact four, or even five, smaller meals a day can keep you trim, and as long as you eat the correct foods then this will help you maintain good energy levels for your surf sessions.

- Start each training session well hydrated. And after exercise aim to drink around 1.5 litres of fluid. Sports drinks provide both carbohydrate and hydration and are useful for intense exercise.
- Start a smart snacking programme. You will mostly likely see high-sugar and high-fat snacks advertised more than the healthy options, so plan out your snacks and give the unhealthy options a wide berth. Good choices are fresh fruit (especially bananas), natural cereal bars, nuts, raisins and oatcakes with hummus or cheese. These are also good pre-surf snacks, as they will keep your energy levels up during your session. Start to refuel as soon as you can after exercise.
- Avoid sugary foods. Sugar is turned into glucose very quickly, which gives you an energy spike then leaves you feeling hungry sooner than after healthy snacks. If you crave sweet stuff, try a few squares of dark chocolate and curb your temptations!
- If it's cold, think about making flasks of warm drinks like hot blackcurrant or potato-based soups for after your surf. It helps your body recover quicker.
- Eat green veg rather than starchy foods with your evening meal. You're likely to be less active later in the day so you won't need quick-release energy, but rather the slower release energy you'll get from these complex carbs.
- If it's late at night, eating baked beans is better than not eating at all!

Stay 'Surf Trim'

A good mixture of exercises is needed to stay surf trim, and it's important to combine steady aerobic training with some high intensity workouts.
During a high intensity workout, or paddling out in a heavy swell, a lot of your energy will come from glycogen – sugars stored in the liver and muscle fibres. However, for the lower intensity surf or workout, most of your energy will come from fat stores.

Why do we store fat?
Otherwise known as adipose tissue, fat is found all over the body and it acts as an insulator from the cold. The body also stores fats around internal organs to help give them protection.

Fat metabolism and energy release
The fat tissue is made up mostly of lipid-filled fat cells known as adiposities, which are stuck together with collagen fibres. These are energy rich and start to activate energy release when the glycogen starts to deplete. Once additional energy is required, the fats can be released from the tissue by a process known as lipolysis.

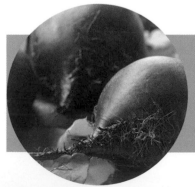

Beetroot Juice Boosts Endurance

beetroot juice can boost stamina and could help people exercise (and surf) for up to 16% longer. Nitrate contained in the vegetable leads to a reduction in oxygen uptake - making exercise less tiring. Beetroot juice reduces VO2 levels during moderate intensity exercise.

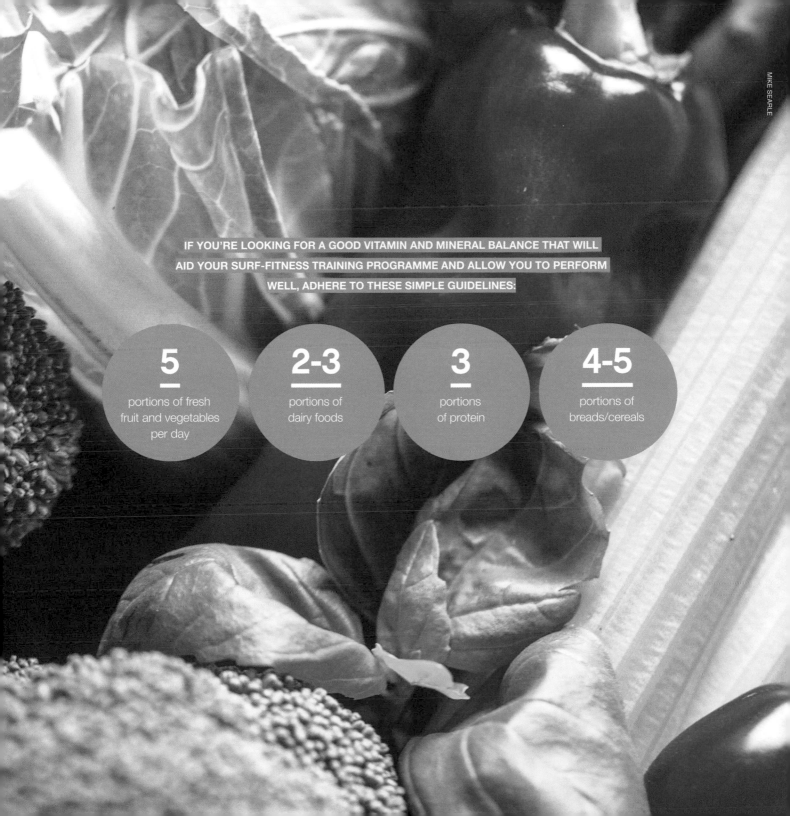

IF YOU'RE LOOKING FOR A GOOD VITAMIN AND MINERAL BALANCE THAT WILL
AID YOUR SURF-FITNESS TRAINING PROGRAMME AND ALLOW YOU TO PERFORM
WELL, ADHERE TO THESE SIMPLE GUIDELINES:

5

portions of fresh
fruit and vegetables
per day

2-3

portions of
dairy foods

3

portions
of protein

4-5

portions of
breads/cereals

CLEAR SKIN · FIT BODY · TONED MUSCLES
BIG SMILE!

Are you getting enough vitamins in your diet?

Believe it or not, our bodies only really need a small amount of vitamins and minerals to function well, keep illness away, and support brain function, the immune system and the nervous system.

Here's a basic breakdown of each vitamins function and where you can find it.

vitamins...

VITAMIN	FUNCTION	SOURCE
Vitamin A	Good eyes, skin and healthy bones	Milk, butter, eggs, dark green veg, dark fruits
Beta carotene	Helps prevent infections	Fruit and vegetables
B1 Thiamine	Used in energy breakdown, healthy nerves	Meat, nuts, most whole grains
B2 Riboflavin	Healthy skin, supports vision	Dairy products, dark green veg, whole grains
B3 Niacin	Used in energy release	Meat, milk, eggs, meat fish, whole grains
Vitamin 12	Building blocks of new cells	Meat, milk, eggs, fish,
Folic acid	Helps form new cells	Liver, green veg, beans, nuts
Vitamin C	Antioxidant, helps fight infection	Citrus fruit, broccoli, tomatoes, melons, dark green veg
Vitamin D	Strong bones and teeth	Milk, eggs, liver
Vitamin E	Antioxidant, aids cell development	Vegetable oils, green veg
Vitamin K	Aids blood clotting	Green leafy veg, cabbage, liver

and minerals...

MINERAL	FUNCTION	SOURCE
Calcium	Strong bones, teeth, muscle contraction, blood and nerve function	Milk, green veg, salmon, shrimps, some fruit juice
Chloride	Good fluid balance	Salt, processed foods
Chromium	Aids energy release	Meat, whole grains, veg oil
Fluoride	Formation of the bones and teeth	Water and toothpaste
Iodine	Helps the production of thyroid hormone	Iodised salt and seafoods
Iron	Helps with the production of haemoglobin, which carries oxygen round the body	Red meat, eggs, some breads, green veg, some dried fruit
Magnesium	Helps develop good bones and teeth	Meat, eggs, some breads, green veg, nuts
Sodium	Aids good fluid balance	Found in many foods
Sulphur	Part of protein and thiamine	Protein-rich foods
Zinc	Helps activate enzymes	Meat, poultry, fish

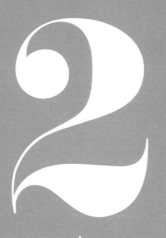

2

get surf fit

SURFING IS A DEMANDING SPORT. THIS RANGE OF EXERCISES WILL IMPROVE YOUR PERFORMANCE – FROM PADDLING OUT TO BUSTING OUT MOVES AT YOUR LOCAL BREAK. THESE FITNESS PROGRAMMES WILL MAKE YOU STRONGER, FITTER AND FASTER, AND CAN BE DONE ANYWHERE FROM YOUR HOME TO THE GYM.

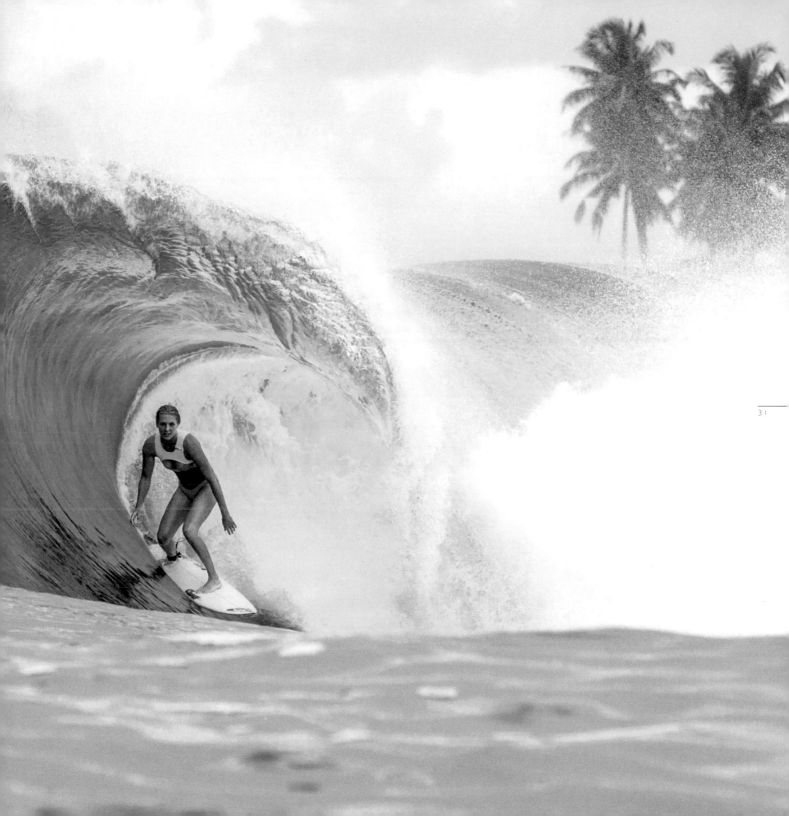

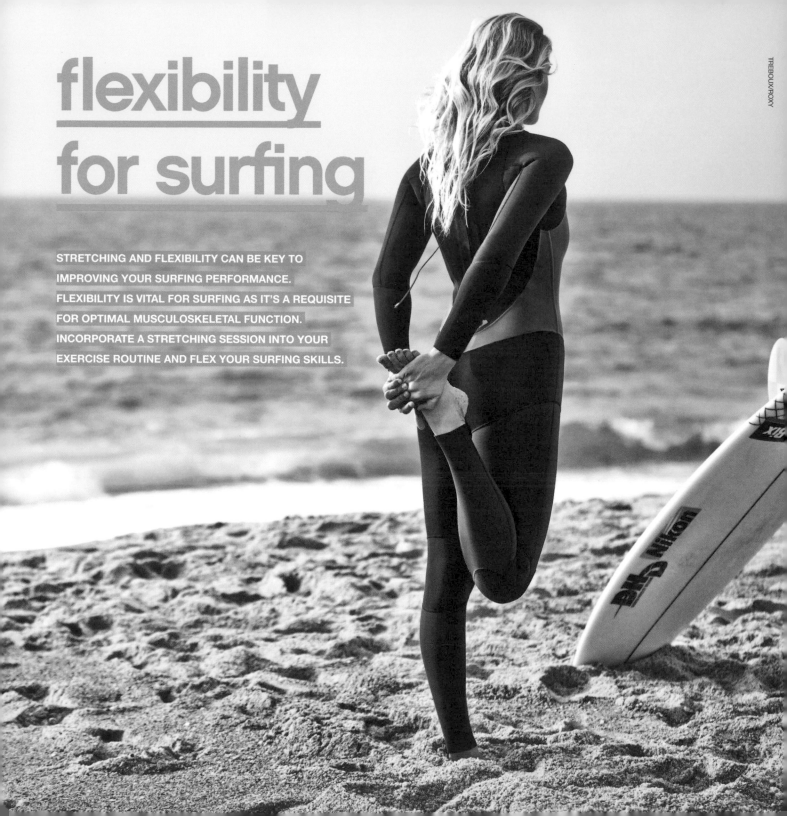

flexibility
for surfing

STRETCHING AND FLEXIBILITY CAN BE KEY TO
IMPROVING YOUR SURFING PERFORMANCE.
FLEXIBILITY IS VITAL FOR SURFING AS IT'S A REQUISITE
FOR OPTIMAL MUSCULOSKELETAL FUNCTION.
INCORPORATE A STRETCHING SESSION INTO YOUR
EXERCISE ROUTINE AND FLEX YOUR SURFING SKILLS.

Types of stretching

There are various stretching techniques that can be used to maintain, and increase, flexibility for surfing.

warming up

• Pre-stretches

Help prepare the muscles for the forthcoming activity, thus reducing the risk of injury and enhancing performance.

Pre-stretches are usually performed after a warm up, targeting the muscle groups to be used in the exercise session. These are light stretches that should be held at a point of mild tension for around 10 seconds.

• Dynamic

Using controlled, rhythmic, repeated movement to take a joint through its normal range of movement (ROM) to the point of tension and back.

For example, from a seated position, extend one leg in front of you and draw the toes towards the knee (dorsal-flexion) until tension is felt, return to full toe point (plantar-flexion) and repeat 10 times.

Each motion should take at least three seconds. Using controlled movements, this type of stretching also lubricates the joints by stimulating the production of synovial fluid.

The combination of light activity and joint lubrication is known as mobilisation, and is perfect for warming up for the many movements in surfing.

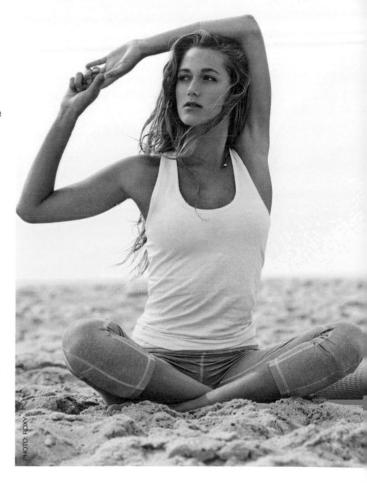

cooling down

• Maintenance stretches

Performed post exercise or surf session, targeting the muscles used to return them to their pre-exercise length, thus maintaining the available ROM (range of movement), reducing soreness and aiding recovery. Typically, they are held at a point of mild tension for approximately 10-20 seconds.

• Static

Slowly stretching a muscle through its range to a point of mild discomfort/tension and maintaining this lengthened position for a period of up to 60 seconds.

Also known as cool down stretching, static is the most well-known stretching type and can be a safe and effective way of stretching after a surf.

• Passive

Refers to the use of an external force, such as gravity, the use of another limb, or a partner or sports massage practitioner to accomplish a static stretch.

In passive-static stretching the athlete uses a prop to resist a force, in order to extend or deepen a stretch. The prop may be as simple as using hand and arm strength to deepen a hamstring stretch, or a towel hooked over the heel to draw the leg into a deeper hamstring stretch. This type of flexibility training can be highly beneficial to surfers, however it's best done under the guidance of an experienced professional.

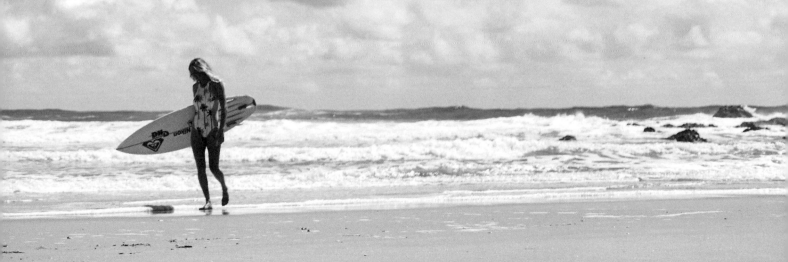

• Active

Promotes a static stretch at the extension of the antagonist muscle, by activating an isometric contraction (where force is exerted but muscle length does not change) at the full inner position of the joint.

For example, fully contracting the hamstrings to full knee flexion will encourage a mechanical stretch of the quadriceps, which will be enhanced by reciprocal inhibition. This type of stretching is useful for dancers and martial artists, or others who need strength at extreme ranges of motion.

• Ballistic

Rapid, bouncy, repeated movements beyond normal ROM with a slow return to the start position.

This is the most controversial form of stretching, as abnormal stretch reflexes can cause damage to the muscles unit or associated joint structures. Necessary only in sport-specific instances where muscle is at risk of injury in explosive activities, it is often incorporated into the routines of sprinters, hurdlers and martial artists. With this in mind this is not a good form of stretching for surfers.

• Developmental stretches

Generally performed at the end of a training session or on a separate occasion after a considerable warm up, and used to lengthen the targeted muscles.

Although there are various ways in which developmental stretches can be performed, essentially there are two phases:
A muscle is slowly stretched to a point of mild tension/discomfort and held in this position for around 6-10 seconds; this should be sufficient time for the stretch reflex to ease off. At this point, the tension in the muscle should have reduced, allowing the muscle to be stretched a little further.

These phases can be repeated several times, with the entire process lasting approximately 30 seconds.

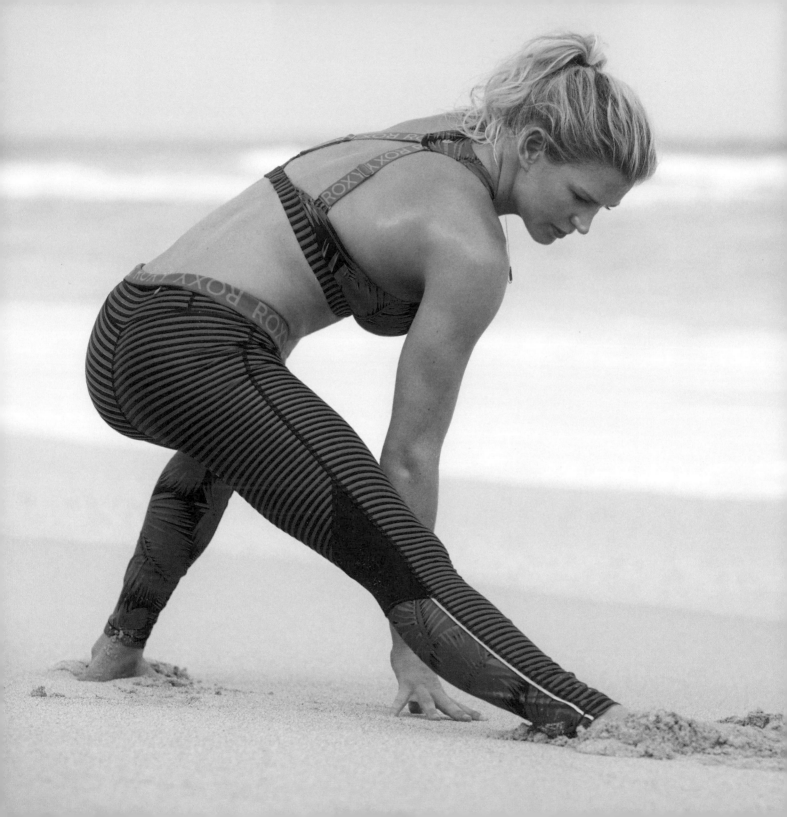

when to stretch

Should I stretch before surfing? As a basic rule, try not to overstretch before any exercise or hitting the water. Some light stretching can be done, but it may be better to mobilise joints and ligaments and warm up muscles before any Intense stretching session.

Guidelines for Stretching

- All stretches should be taught and performed in a slow and controlled manner, ensuring participants can facilitate the most effective stretch and reduce the risk of injury.
- For best results, stretching should be done on a regular basis.
- It is very important to stretch to a point of mild tension/discomfort, and never stretch to the point of pain.
- If you are not sure of a particular stretching technique then you should consult a trained professional.
- Stretches aimed at developing flexibility should be undertaken with care (especially with young surfers) and held for about 30 seconds.
- Try to breathe normally while stretching and try to exhale when initiating a developmental stretch.
- Always aim for a well-balanced stretching programme. During surfing sessions and movements many muscle groups are used, with the upper body, torso and pelvic areas being used widely.
- Always ensure a thorough warm up is performed prior to stretching.
- Poor stretching techniques can lead to injury.

When shouldn't I stretch?

- If there is, or has recently been (in the last 3 days), an injury to the targeted muscle.
- If a joint is infected or inflamed.
- If a sharp pain is felt in the muscle or joint.
- If you are unsure of a particular stretch don't try it: seek advice!

Basic Stretching

01. Arm Raises

- Start with your arms in front.
- As you take a slow, deep breath in, raise your hands over your head and stretch backwards.
- As you slowly breathe out, lower your arms.
- Gradually enlarge the circles, as you repeat.
- Repeat 3 - 5 times.

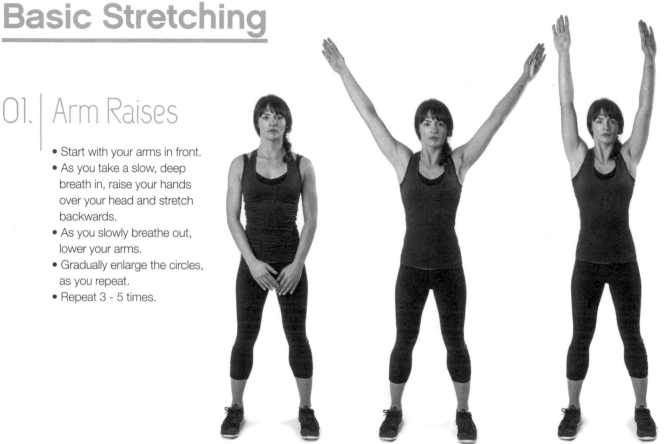

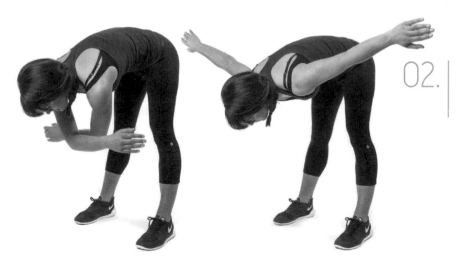

02. Bent-Over Arm Swings

Again this is an area for major consideration, if you're keen to paddle out back faster, then this area of mobility is key.

- Stand with your feet about a hip-width apart with soft knees.
- Lean forwards and let your arms hang downwards, then swing your arms so that you reach backwards to slap your back.
- Repeat 10 times.

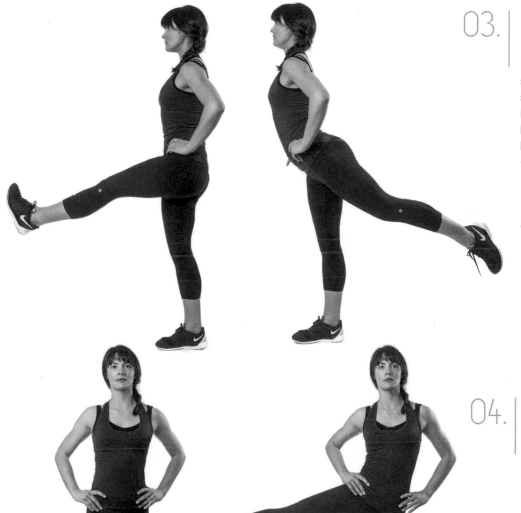

03. | Leg Swings

Many surfers will get a groin strain at some point. This simple leg exercise can help in this area by warming up the hip flexors and preparing your body for that first pop up.

- Relax your left leg and simply let it swing backwards and forwards 10 times before repeating on the other side.
- You may need the support of a partner for this.

04. | Leg Swing Cross Over

This is another great exercise for warming up hip flexors and preparing for pop ups.

- Relax and swing your leg across your body line to the left before swinging back to the starting position.
- Do this 10 times before repeating on the other side.
- Again, you may need support for this.

05. | Basic Arm Swings

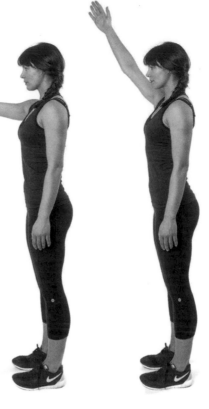
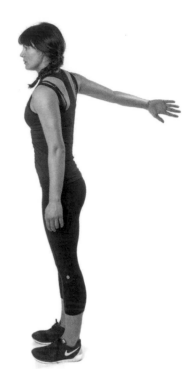

A simple but effective light exercise that will get you ready for a paddle out.

- Standing with your feet hip-width apart and facing forwards.
- With relaxed arms swing your left arm forwards 10 times before repeating on the other side.
- After this, reverse the movement.

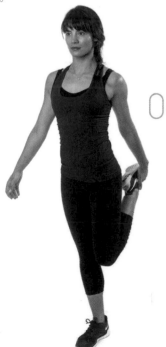

06. | Quad Stretch

The quadriceps are the largest muscle group in the body and can be stretched in many ways.

- Try a simple stand on one leg with knees together. Slowly pull your foot upwards towards the buttocks and hold for 20 seconds, then repeat.
- If you're a little wobbly then hold a wall or a training partner.

07. | Hamstring Stretch

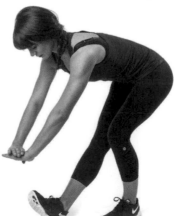

- Slowly lean forwards with one leg slightly bent and one leg extended forwards.
- Hold for 10 seconds.

08. | Spinal Mobility Twists

A great mobility exercise for the muscles of the spine.

• With feet pointing forwards, slowly twist from side to side.

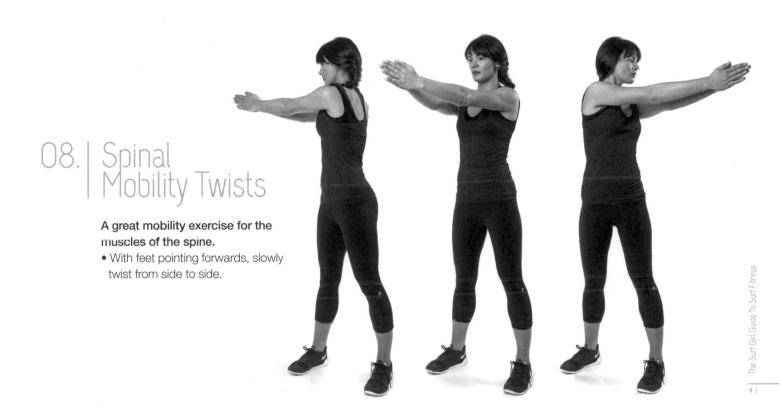

Why are we warming up?

As you prepare your body to surf it's important to think about just what you are warming up: ligaments, tendons and muscles sending rich oxygenated blood to the vital areas so that your paddle out (and your first few waves) are done with the least amount of effort.

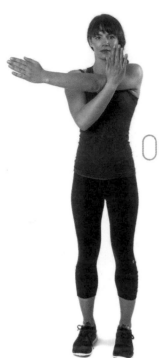

09. | Shoulder Stretch

- Start with both feet pointing forwards.
- Take one arm across the body and lightly press on the back of the arm; avoid pressing on any joints.

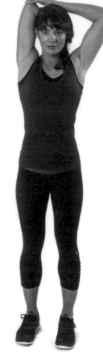

10. | Tricep Stretch

- Start with knees soft, pointing forward, feet about hip-width apart.
- Take one arm up, keeping it close to the back of the head.
- From here slowly press lightly downwards on the elbow, feeling a light stretch on the back of the arm.
- Hold for 20 seconds, then repeat on the other side.

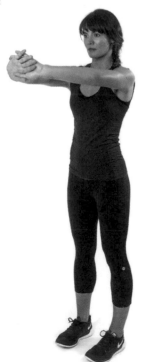

11. | Upper Back Stretch

- Stand with feet about hip width apart.
- Clasp your hands out in front of you so that you feel a nice stretch through the shoulder blades.
- Hold the stretch for 10 seconds then repeat 3-4 times.

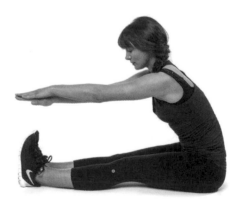

12. | Sit and Reach Stretch

- Start by sitting on the floor with both legs out in front, then slowly reach forward to touch your toes – this will stretch the hamstrings and the spine.
- Aim for a smooth and controlled movement.

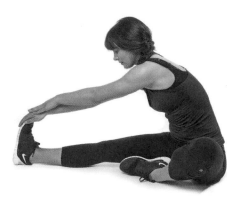

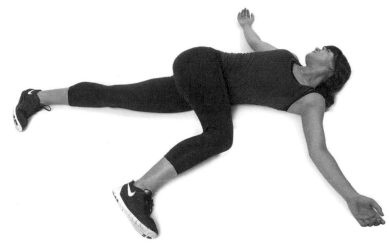

13. | Hamstring Stretch 2

Tight hamstrings can be painful and, as a surfer, taking care of this area is highly important.
- Start the stretch by sitting with your right leg straight and your left leg bent.
- Slowly reach forward with the right hand and grip the bottom of your foot, keeping the leg still and extended by lightly pressing on your knee.

14. | Gluteal Stretch

The gluteal muscles play a major role in surfing movements and can often become tight.
- Lying on the floor with one leg extended, try flexing the other leg.
- As you do pull it upwards and across towards your shoulder area.

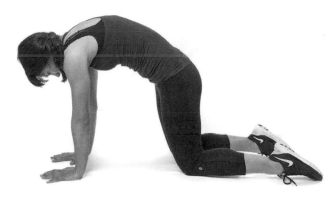

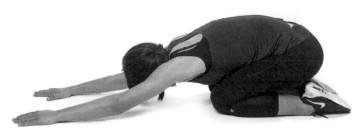

15. | Cat Stretch

A great stretch for your back.
- Start the exercise on hands and knees, and from here pull your tummy inwards, and slowly arch your back, hold for 20+ seconds then repeat.

16. | Thoracic Extension Stretch

This should give your lats and back a good stretch.
- Start on your knees, place hands on floor and reach forwards.
- Hold for 10 seconds.

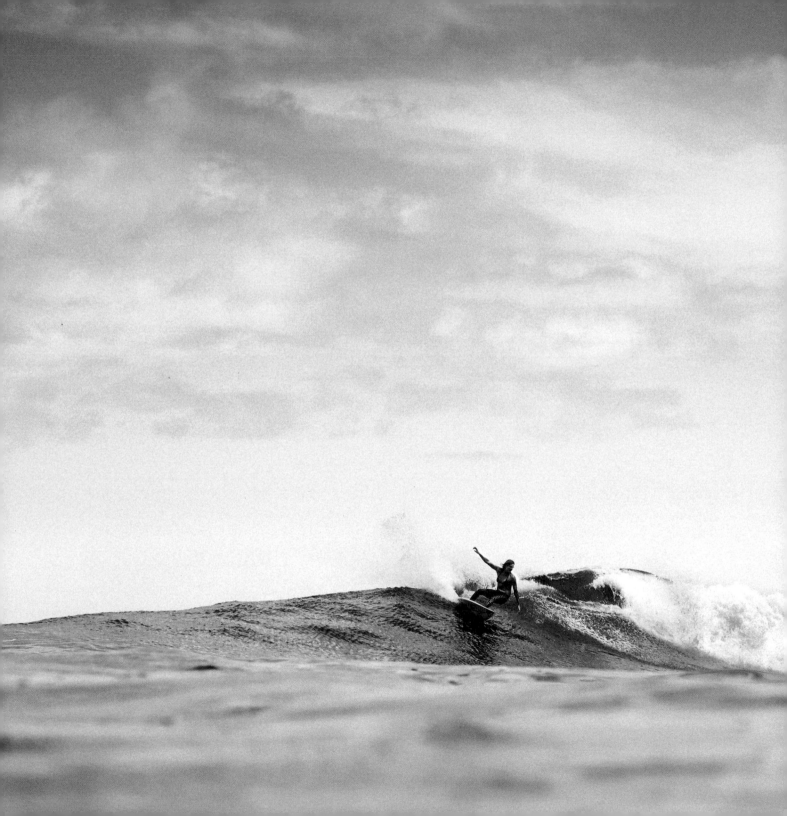

FOCUS

power to the
core

Strengthening your Core

So much emphasis is put on "Core Training", whether it's for general fitness, rehabilitation or sport performance. Why? Because it's your body's foundation for movement, power, stabilization and protection... So, a poor core impedes your fitness, and can leave you wide open to injury. In surfing terms, a strong core enables you to improve your power, performance and stability, which will help you to both catch the wave of your life and ride it down the line with coordinated style!

WHAT'S CORE STABILITY TRAINING?

A great way to start if you're looking at undertaking a new exercise programme, core stability training focuses on the muscles at the heart of all the body's movements.

The aim of core training is to increase the efficiency of the smaller, deeper, stabilising muscles that help you balance. The muscles of the abdominal area and torso help stabilise the spine and provide a solid foundation for many surfing moves.

Core training is cost-free and can be done anywhere, at any time. Exercises range in difficulty from beginner to advanced. As you progress you can integrate the use of various equipment to increase your core strength.

If you are new to core stability training it is vital to take it one step at a time and avoid any exercises that you are unsure of or cause you pain.

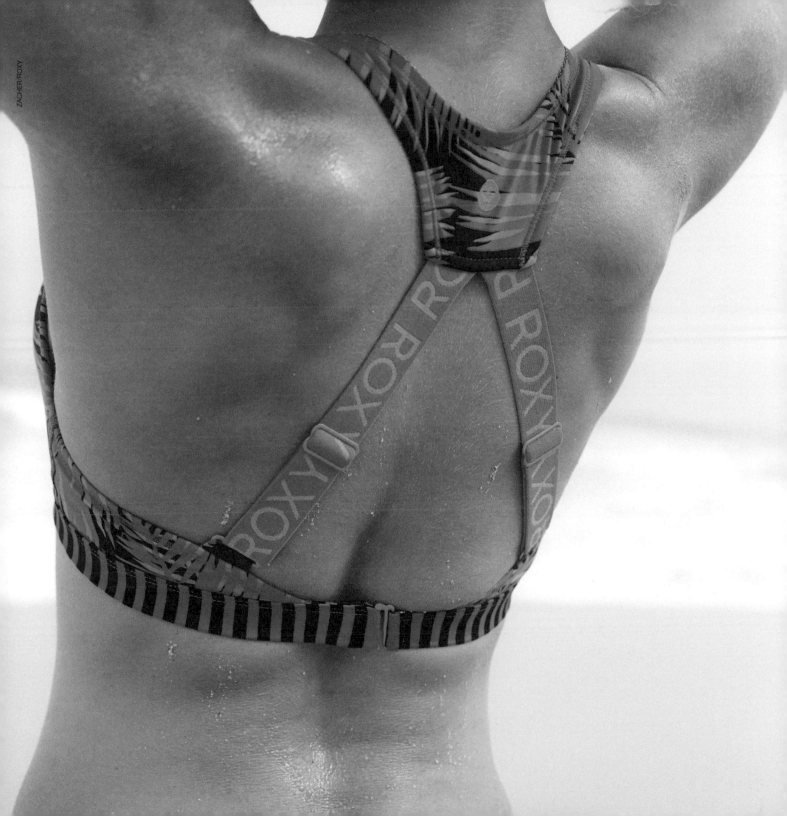

abs and obliques

01. | Basic Crunch

This will strengthen your abdominals.
- Start by placing your hands on your thighs, then simply run your hands upwards towards your knees.
- Then lower slowly back down again before repeating.

How many? Try 10 reps.

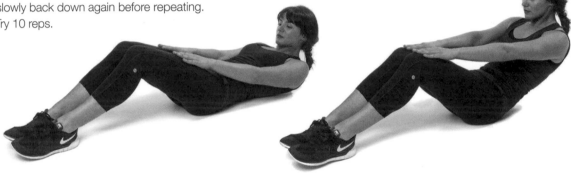

02. | Russian Twist

A great exercise that is used to work the abdomen muscles.
- Start by sitting on the floor with your hips and knees bent 90 degrees.
- Hold the weight straight out in front of you and keep your back straight.
- Twist your torso as far as you can to the left, and then reverse the motion, twisting as far as you can to the right. That's one rep.

How many? Try 3 sets of 8.

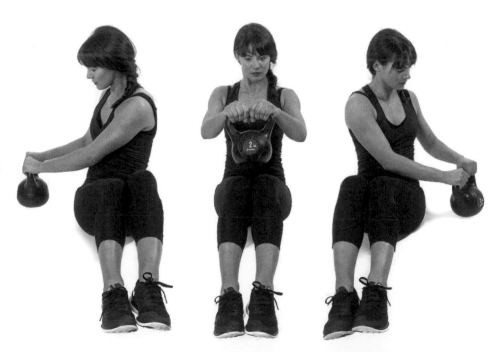

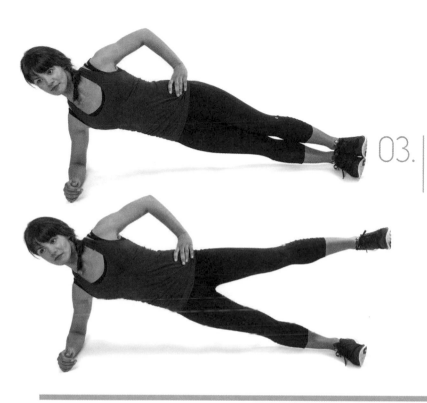

03. | Side Plank with Leg Raise

- Start in the side plank position.
- Once you are in the correct position lift one leg upward, a few inches off from the other one, and hold.

How many? Hold for 10 seconds then change sides.

How will core strength benefit my surfing?

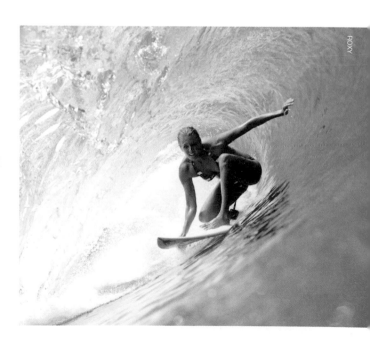

ROXY

- Greater efficiency of movement.
- Improved body control and balance.
- Increased power output from both the core musculature and peripheral muscles such as the shoulders, arms and legs.
- Reduced risk of injury.
- Improved balance and stability.
- Improved surfing performance.

TOP TIP

Your spine should always be in a neutral position – one where your lower back is naturally curved, not flattened or arched. This will put your pelvis in a stress-free position and activate your abdominals, particularly your transverse abdominals.

04. | Side Plank Star Position with Leg Raise

- Start the exercise on your side with legs extended, supporting your body on your forearm and keeping your head in line with the spine.
- From this position shift your weight onto your hand, whilst raising your hip off the floor and extending your other arm upwards.

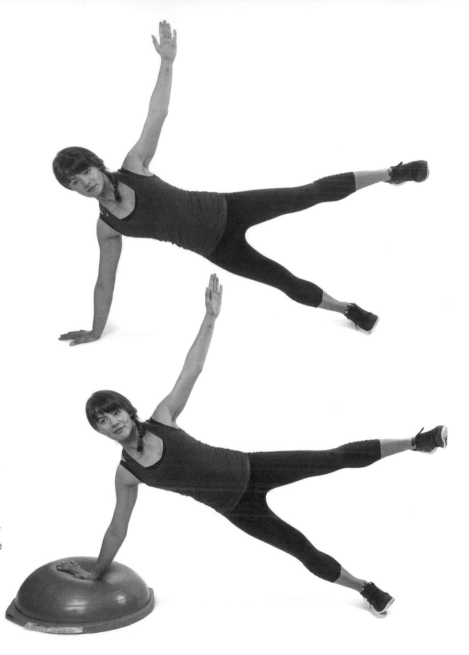

05. | Side Plank Star Position using BOSU

For this advanced exercise you will need a Bosu Balance Trainer or an Indo Board with Gigante cushion.

- Start the exercise in the same way as before, only this time place one hand on the centre of the Bosu Balance Trainer.
- The added challenge will come with the instability of the Bosu or Indo Board.

SUMMARY {
- Always maintain a good posture.
- Core training can be done every day.
- If you suffer from back problems some core exercises might not be suitable - always consult a doctor if you're unsure.
- Always work within your capabilities.
}

06. | Crunch with twist

- Lay flat on your back with hands behind your head.
- Contract your lower abs to raise your legs a few inches off the ground.
- Twist your torso and bend your left knee so that your right elbow crosses your body and reaches toward your left knee.
- Switch and twist to the other side so that your left elbow reaches toward your bent right knee.
- Continue alternating sides without tucking your chin toward your chest.

the plank

Great to increase your power and stability for paddling, plank exercises will strengthen your abdominals, back and shoulders – specifically your transverse abdominals, which are the deepest layer of abdominal muscles that wrap around your mid-section.

01. | Front Plank

- Position yourself so that your toes are on the ground and your elbows are directly below your shoulders, then raise yourself up, keeping a straight line from your shoulders to your ankles, so that your elbows and toes support your body.
- Use your tummy muscles to maintain the position, keep your head in line with your spine and try not to stick your bottom in the air.

How many? Try 4 x 30 seconds for starters

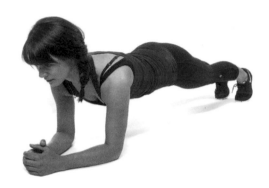

02. | Front Plank (with ball) in Press-up Position

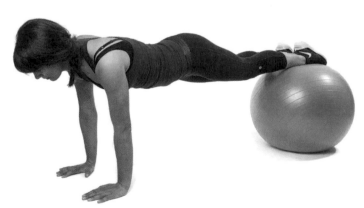

This version is slightly trickier than the ordinary plank.
- Start by draping your body over the ball, placing your palms flat on the floor in front of you, and extending your legs straight out behind you.
- Slowly walk your hands forward until the ball is beneath your shins. Keep your legs together and point your toes. Align your shoulders with your wrists and spread your fingers wide apart for support.
- Maintain good spinal alignment: keep your back straight and in line with your head. If your belly is sagging then you're not engaging your core properly.
- Shoulders should be kept in line with the wrists.
- Hold this position with the tummy muscles tight and contract your abs to make a flat surface.

How many? Try 4 x 15 seconds and as you get stronger hold for longer.

03. | Swiss Ball Plank

• Start this exercise with elbows on the Swiss ball, keep your head in line with your spine, legs slightly apart and use your arms to support your body. Hold the position.

04. | Front Plank with Leg Lift (with Gigante)

• Start this exercise in the same way as the basic plank, only this time try lifting one foot off the ground, just for a few seconds, to overload your core and then swap to the other side.

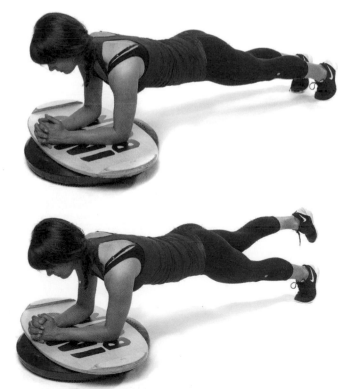

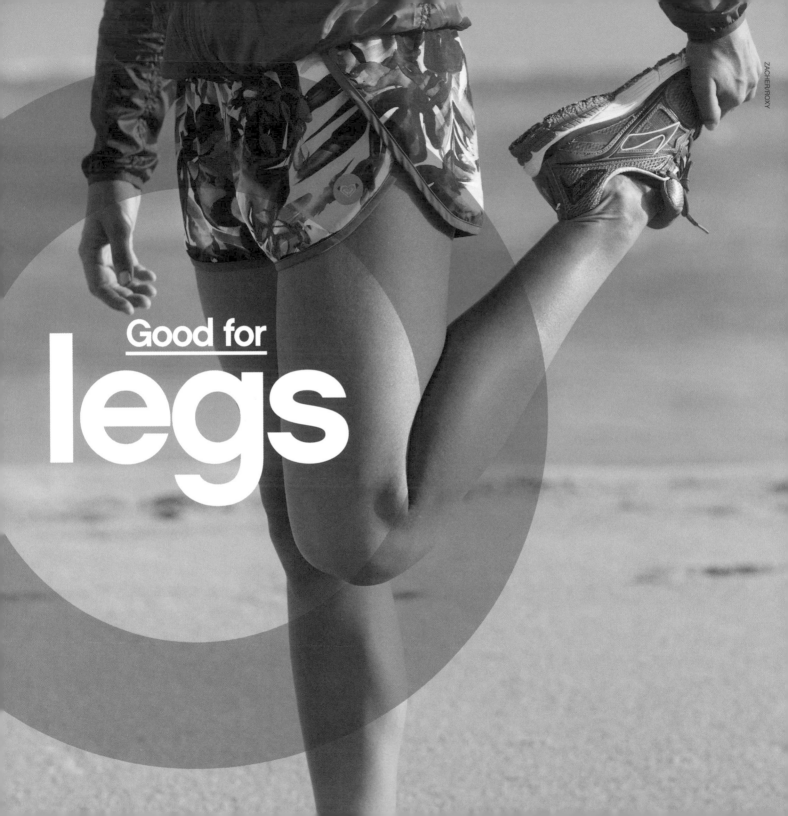

Good for
legs

lunges

Once you get past the beginner stage, movements on a surfboard can be difficult and leg strength is vital for sharp turns and board movement. A basic weights workout incorporating lunges and steps can really benefit your surfing and is great for improving the hamstrings, quadriceps, buttocks, balance and general leg strength.

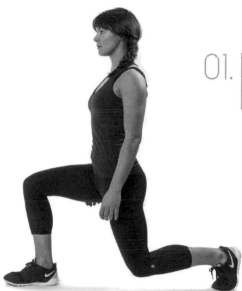

01. | Lunge

- Start the exercise with hands by your sides, shoulders back.
- Step forwards, feet pointing in the same direction, aiming for a 90-degree angle.

How many? Try a few to get your balance, then a basic set could be 4 x 20 seconds non-stop.

02. | Lunge with Weights
(STATIC)

- Start the exercise with weights by your sides, shoulders back.
- Step forwards, feet pointing in the same direction, aiming for a 90-degree angle.

How many? Try a few to get your balance, then a basic set could be 4 x 20 seconds non-stop.

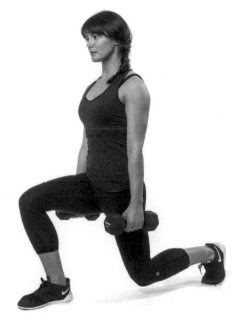

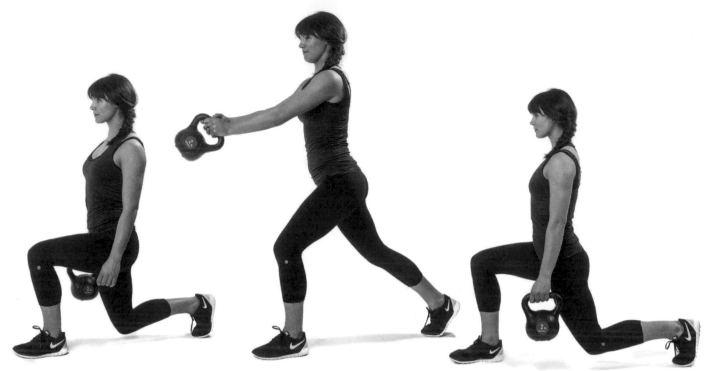

03. | Lunge with Kettlebell (WALKING)

- Start the exercise with the kettlebell in your left hand, shoulders back, in a lunge postion.
- Walk forwards and during the forward motion, swing the kettlebell to your front and swap hands.
- Lower your body back to the lunge position with the kettlebell in the opposite hand.

How many? Try 4 x 5/6 steps, then rest.

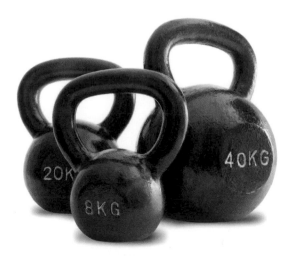

Kettlebells

These cast iron or steel weights (which look a bit like a cannonball with a handle) are used to perform ballistic exercises that combine cardiovascular, strength and flexibility training. Perfect for building general strength for surfing fitness, they will also tone and strengthen buttocks, legs, hips, tummies and backs of arms.

04. | Step Lunge with Bicep Curl

- Start the exercise with weights by your sides, shoulders back.
- Keeping your back straight, step forwards and bring your weights up into a biceps curl, keeping your elbows tucked in.
- Slowly, return to the start position, lowering the weights to rest by your sides.

How many? Try 6-8 reps, then rest.

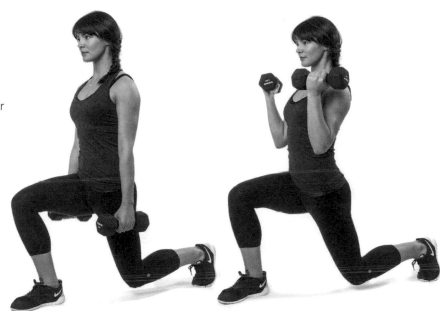

05. | BOSU Single Leg Balance

- To strengthen your ankles and knees try standing on the Bosu Balance Trainer with the dome side down.
- Stand in the centre of the deck and raise one foot slightly off the deck whilst maintaining a good upright body posture.
- Hold for 8-10 seconds before changing legs.

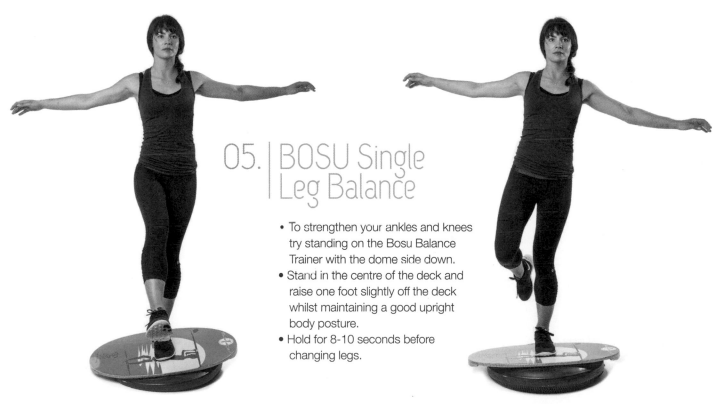

squats

Squats are a full-body fitness staple that work the hamstrings, quadriceps and buttocks, while improving balance, co-ordination and general leg strength. They can be done anywhere in many different ways – you can even do them at home in front of the TV.

01. | Basic Squats

- Start by standing with feet hip-width apart.
- Lower down towards an almost 90-degree angle, keeping your shoulders back. Holding your arms out in front of you will aid balance.

How many? Try 6-8 reps

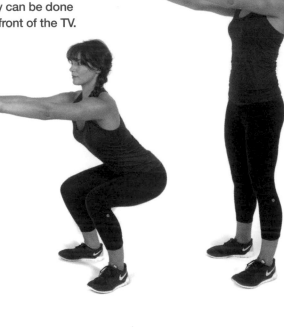

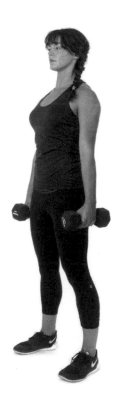

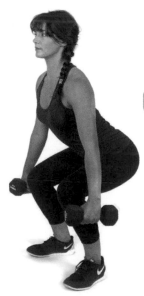

02. | Basic Squats with Weights

- Start by standing with feet hip-width apart.
- Lower down towards an almost 90-degree angle, keeping shoulders back and holding the weights alongside you during the movements.

How many? Try 6-8 reps

03. | Squats with Weights and Front Raise

- Start by standing with feet hip-width apart, holding the weights alongside you.
- Lower down towards an almost 90-degree angle, keeping shoulders back.
- As you squat down, bring the weights up in front of you. As you come up to resting position, lower the weights back down.

How many? Try 6-8 reps

(You may wish to try this exercise without the weights to start with.)

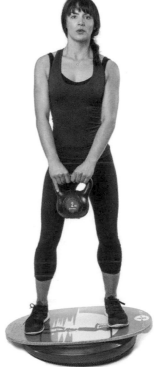
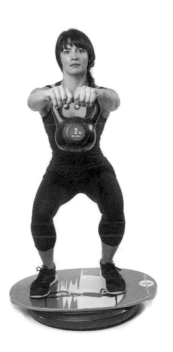

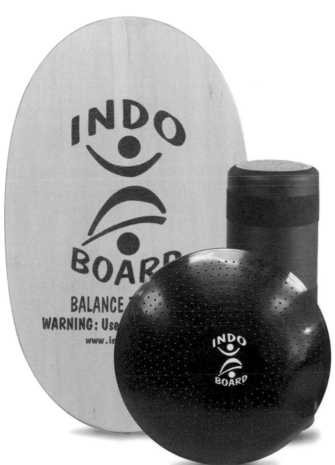

DOING SQUAT THRUSTS ISN'T GOING TO BE ENOUGH ON ITS OWN. TO IMPROVE YOUR SURF FITNESS YOU WILL NEED TO INCORPORATE THEM INTO A WELL BALANCED TRAINING PROGRAMME.

In addition to dynamic leg movements, getting barrelled takes a heightened level of proprioceptive skill (balance). Any balance kit that will allow you to fine tune your backhand can be highly useful.

The Indo board has been around for years. It really is a great bit of kit. Now with the introduction of the Indo Flo Gigante, you can practice your backhand or forehand over and over again.

bosu squats

(slightly more advanced)

A BOSU Balance Trainer (or BOSU ball, as it is often called) is a training device consisting of an inflated rubber hemisphere attached to a rigid platform. Designed to improve balance and strength, it's a great fitness-training tool for surfers.

A BOSU is very wobbly so take care. You may wish to try these exercises without the weights to start with.

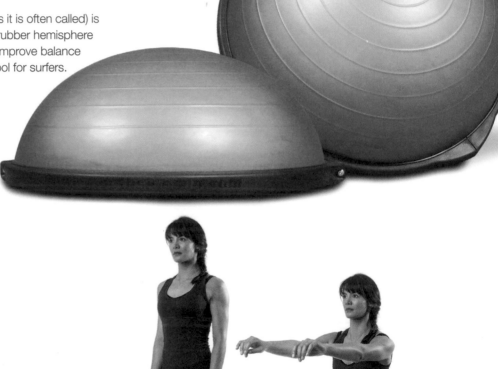

01. | Bosu Squats

- Start with feet hip-width apart on the deck.
- Lower down to an almost 90-degree angle, keeping shoulders back.

How many? Try 6-8 reps

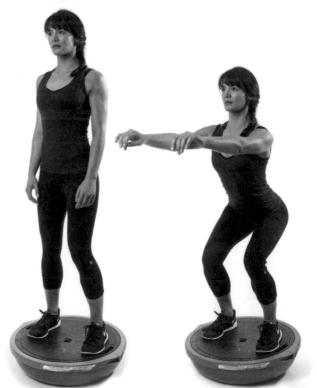

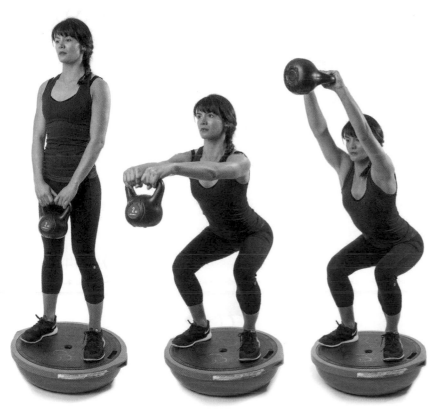

02. | Bosu Squats with Front Raise

- Start with feet hip-width apart on the deck, holding the weights alongside you.
- Lower down to an almost 90-degree angle, keeping shoulders back.
- As you squat down, bring the weights up in front of you. Lower them back down as you return to resting position.

How many? Try 6-8 reps

Whatever leg workout you undertake, try to do a regular 1-2 sessions a week to make a difference. This can be backed up by running, spinning and other cardio gym-based workouts.

JUMP TO IT:
DO POP-UPS EVERYDAY.
AND WHEN YOU FEEL LIKE YOU'VE DONE ENOUGH, DO 10 MORE!

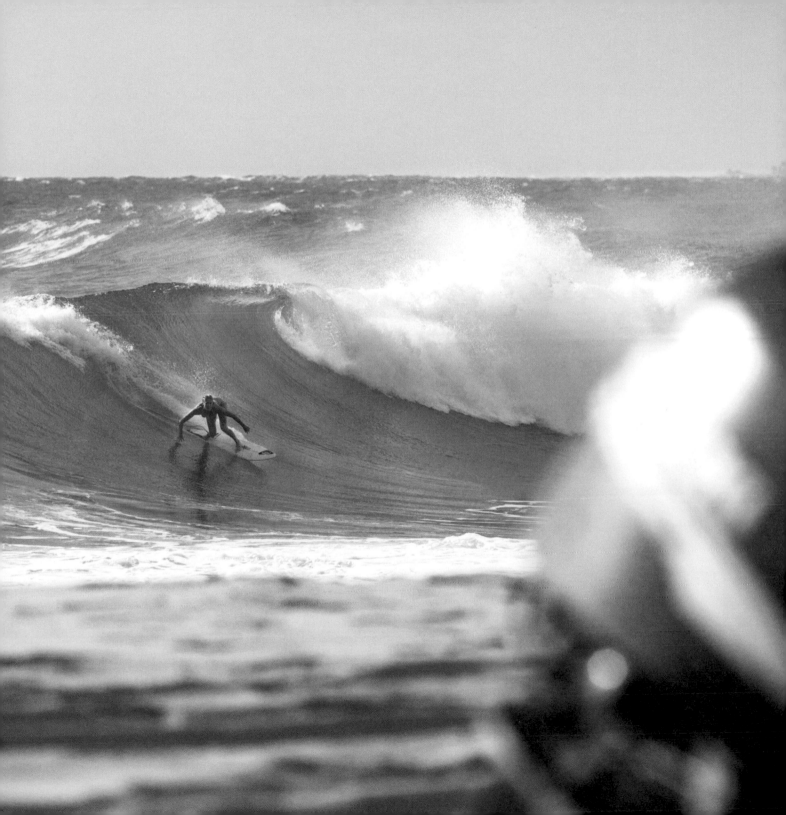

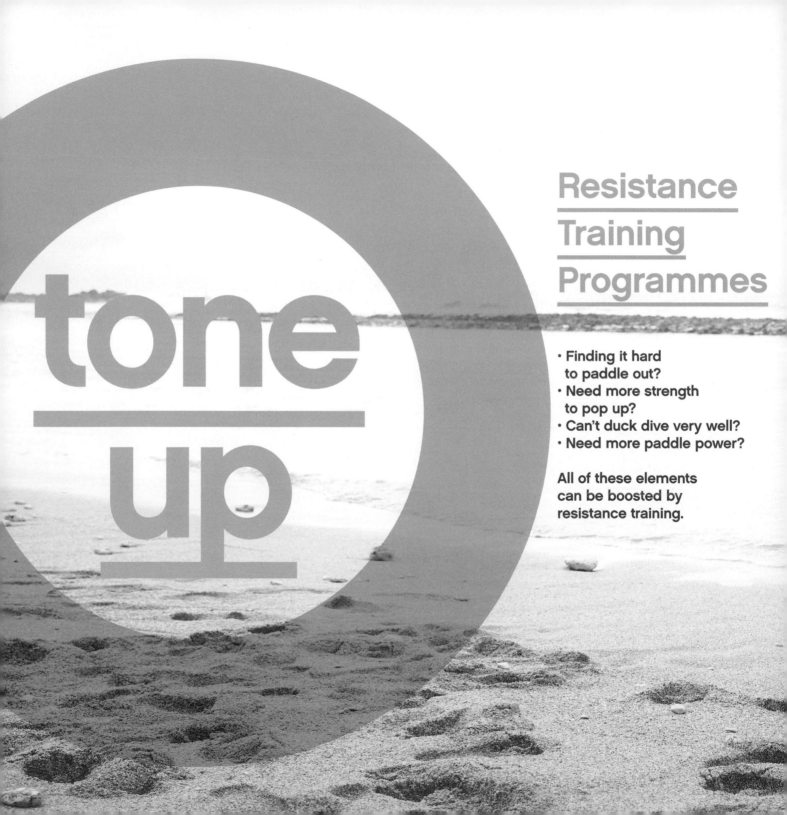

tone up

Resistance Training Programmes

- Finding it hard to paddle out?
- Need more strength to pop up?
- Can't duck dive very well?
- Need more paddle power?

All of these elements can be boosted by resistance training.

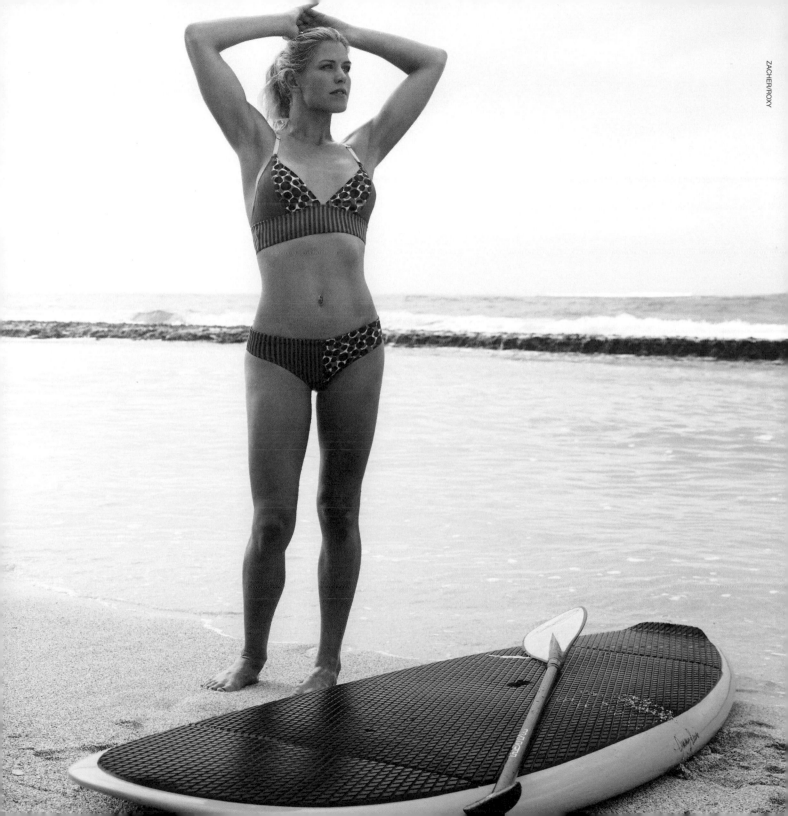

resistance training

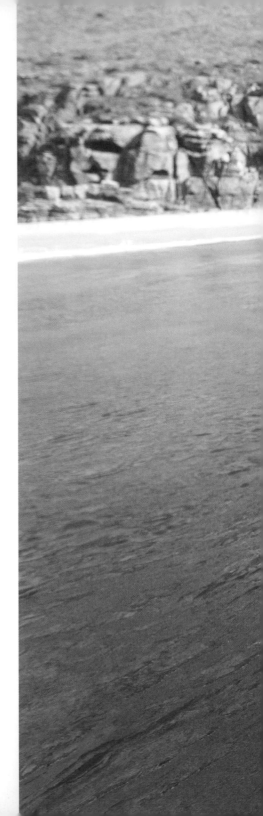

What is resistance training?

Resistance training is simply working out or training with weights – either free weights or on gym machines – by performing simple, repetitive movements that focus on particular muscles.

How much resistance training should I do?

Aim for a well-balanced training programme covering all the major muscle groups, about 2-3 times a week.

It's important to remember that surfing movements demand a lot of flexibility, so lifting too many heavy weights on a regular basis isn't the best workout for a surfer, as it can leave you stiff, with slower dynamic movements. Instead you should adopt a workout that uses light weights and high reps, to build surfing strength and endurance. Incorporate other types of fitness training into your workout and ensure you have a decent stretching programme in place to back up your mobility.

How will resistance training benefit my surfing?

It increases muscle strength and endurance, giving you more stamina and enabling you to put more power behind the explosive movements needed in surfing.

For resistance training to be effective for your surfing, you need to assess what movements you're trying to strengthen and employ exercises that are functional for that move. For example, if your goal is to improve the upper body for improved paddle fitness, you don't want to lift massive weights that could restrict your range of movement (ROM). Instead you would need to focus on endurance strength training – high reps of non-stop exercises that promote strength gains.

Tips for Planning a Resistance Training Programme

- Aim for basic progression and never over train
- Cover all the major muscle groups
- Always use a good technique.
- Use light weights or resistance with high reps
- Train weekly

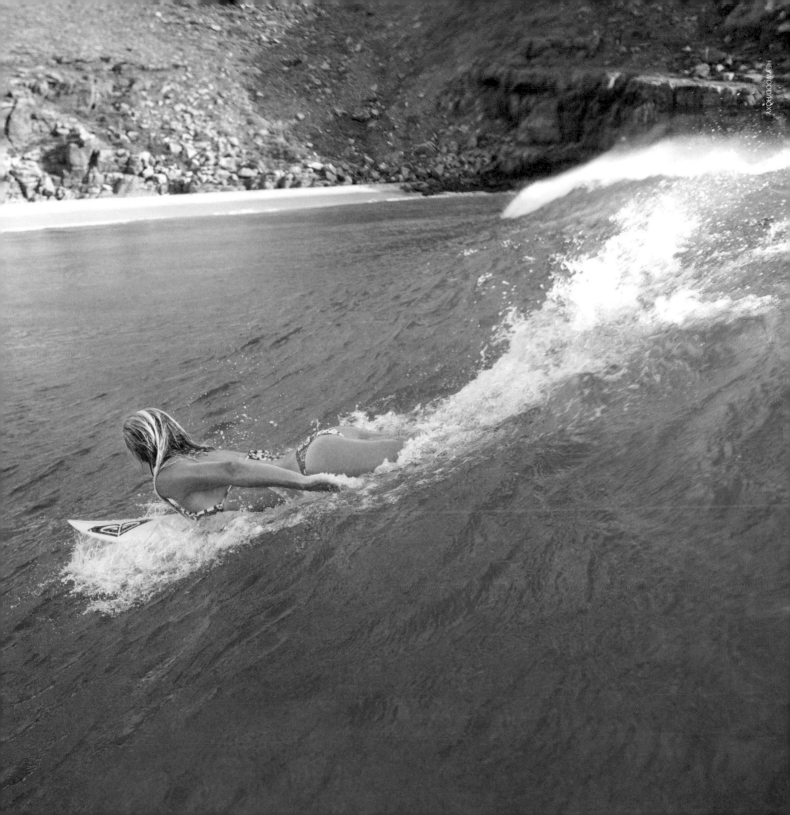

What are the different elements of strength training?

1. Strength Endurance

The more explosive power you start with, the more of it can be maintained for a prolonged period of time. Just like in sports such as distance running, cycling and swimming, in surfing strength endurance can also be vital for performance. Strength endurance can be developed through own bodyweight exercises like pull-ups or press-ups, or the use of light weights and high repetitions.

2. Hypertrophy

Synonymous with most people's perceptions of strength training, hypertrophy refers to increased muscle bulk and size. However, while the likes of football and rugby players require significant bulk to withstand aggressive body contact, for most athletes too much muscle bulk is a hindrance. And remember that a larger muscle is not necessarily a stronger muscle.

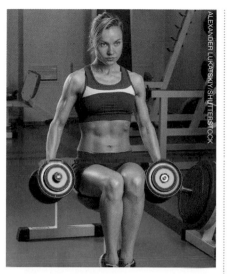

ALEXANDER LUKATSKIY/SHUTTERSTOCK

Strength endurance

Strength endurance can be developed through 'own body weight' exercises like pull ups or press ups, or the use of low weights and high repetitions. again it is important to say that strength training for surfers should not restrict surfing movements and this should be taken into account when designing a surf fitness programme.

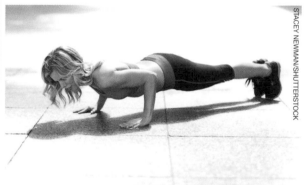

STACEY NEWMAN/SHUTTERSTOCK

3. Explosive Power

This is the key element of strength training for surfers, as dynamic movements are at the heart of surfing performance.

SWILLY

STRENGTH TRAINING WITH YOUR OWN BODY WEIGHT

Using your own body weight for gains in surfing strength can be highly beneficial, and there's no equipment needed. Dips (right) and press ups (above) are great for working the shoulder muscles used for paddling. During surfing movements there are also many demands on the legs; even a basic bottom turn will demand strength and drive from the gluteus maximus (buttocks) for example.

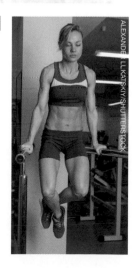

ALEXANDER LUKATSKIY/SHUTTERSTOCK

training kit

Not so long ago a surfer just surfed. These days sports specific training and principles play an important role in improving performance. Regular surfers, landlocked surfers, surfing pros, young surfers and old surfers will all benefit from sports specific training that is tailored to them.

An abundance of kit is available nowadays, but here are some key pieces that are a must for any surfer:

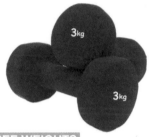

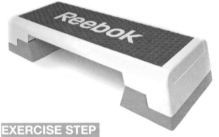

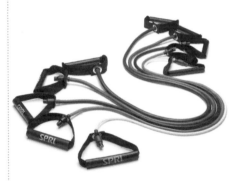

FREE WEIGHTS

Using heavy weights on a regular basis can leave you stiff and slow down your dynamic movements – definitely not something you need if you're a surfer. However, if you adopt a workout using light weights and high reps it will build your surfing strength and endurance so you'll be able to paddle out faster and still have the energy to catch the best waves when it's pumping.

Medicine Ball

Medicine balls (also known as a fitness ball) are highly versatile weighted balls used effectively in plyometric weight training to increase explosive power in athletes in all sports.

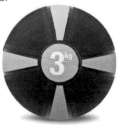

EXERCISE STEP

Height adjustable aerobics steps are versatile pieces of fitness equipment.

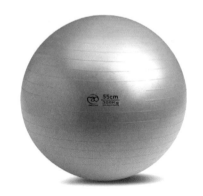

THE SWISS BALL

The Swiss Ball is well know within the global surfing community as it is highly versatile and can be transported easily. Its uses run far and wide, from core strength training to surfing flexibility sessions. Many surfers use them on a regular basis to boost their surfing performance.

RESISTANCE BANDS AND CORDS

As well as using your own body weight for strength training, you can also use different types of resistance bands.

Power Stroke Cords

These can be used for general strength and conditioning, as well as rehabilitation or injury prevention. Resistance band exercises are ideal for home exercise programmes and can easily be incorporated into circuit training to condition the cardiovascular system as well as strengthening specific muscle groups. Because resistance tubing is so compact and light weight, it can also easily be taken away on trips too.

Basic Weight Training

With any Weights Programme some key points should be taken into consideration:

- **Age** If you are under 15 try to use own body weight exercises or resistance bands, and avoid lifting weights.
- **Plan out your session** Look at an all over body programme, a well balanced programme is key to overall fitness and strength gains.

- **Eat after your work out** It is easy to forget to eat properly after training, try not to – a protein shake or cereal bar will keep you going until you have your next main meal.
- **Drink** Don't forgot that drinking during and after your workout is very important.
- **Rest** Over training can take place if you do

not take at least one day off a week.
- **Warm up** Warm up and cool down for 5 to 10 minutes. Walking/jogging is a good way to warm up, then some mobility and stretching is an excellent way to cool down.

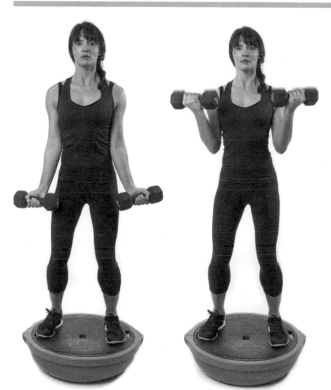

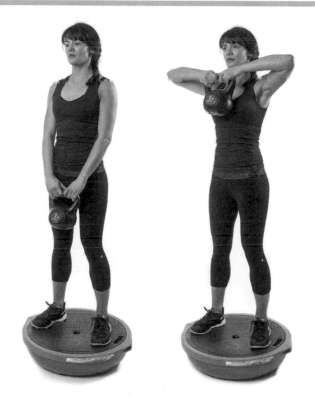

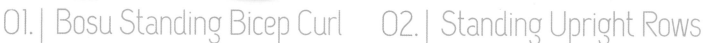

01. | Bosu Standing Bicep Curl

- Stand carefully on the BOSU with feet apart.
- Tuck elbows in, curl the weight upwards, then slowly lower.
How many? Try 8-10 reps then repeat.

02. | Standing Upright Rows

- Start with feet hips-width apart with weights in hands.
- Pull your elbows upwards, keeping the weights close to your body, then repeat.
How many? 8-10 reps.

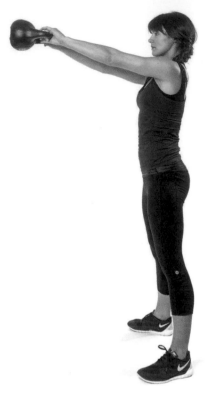
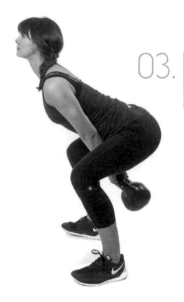

03. | Kettlebell Squats

- Stand with feet apart, facing forwards.
- Slowly squat down and as you do swing the bell between your legs.

How many? Try 10-12 swings before resting.

04. | Basic Swiss Ball Triceps Drop

- Start again on the ball, feet apart. Taking great care with the weight, squeeze the elbows together before lowering down behind your head.
- With the weight lightly resting on the neck extend the weight upwards taking care NOT to lock the elbows to much.

How many? 8-10 reps then repeat

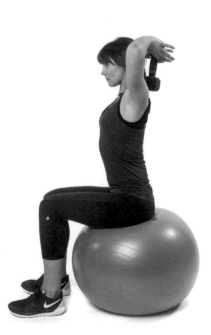
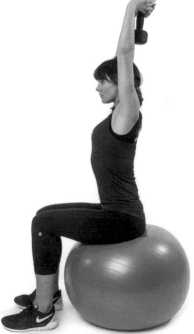

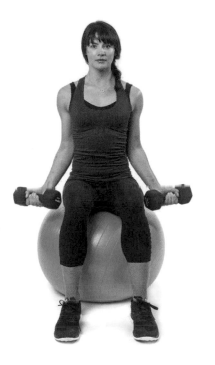
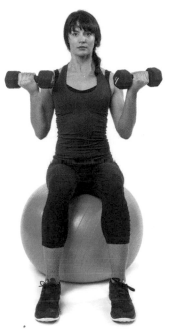

05. | Seated Swiss Ball Shoulder Press from Bicep Curl

- Aim for a good upright body position on the ball, feet about hip-width apart.
- Slowly, with elbows locked in against your body, perform a bicep curl.
- From here push the weights upwards into a shoulder press. Keep your core tight during the movement. Lower and repeat.

How many? 8-10 reps then repeat

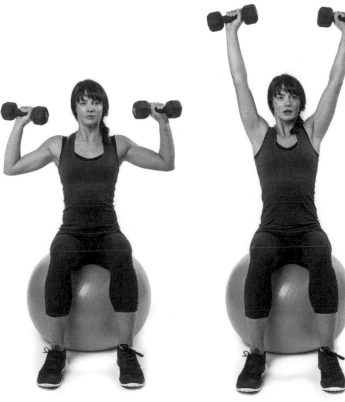

Using Weights

How do I use weights to make me stronger for surfing?

A muscle will only strengthen when forced to operate beyond its customary intensity (overload). Overload can be progressed by increasing:

1. Resistance – the amount of weight lifted
2. Number of repetitions with a particular weight
3. Number of sets of the exercise

Light weights, High Reps

If you want to tone up and increase your strength endurance for surfing, it's important to remember that light to intermediate weights should be used along with high repetition sets (around 15-30).

FLEXIBILITY

COORDINATION

STAMINA

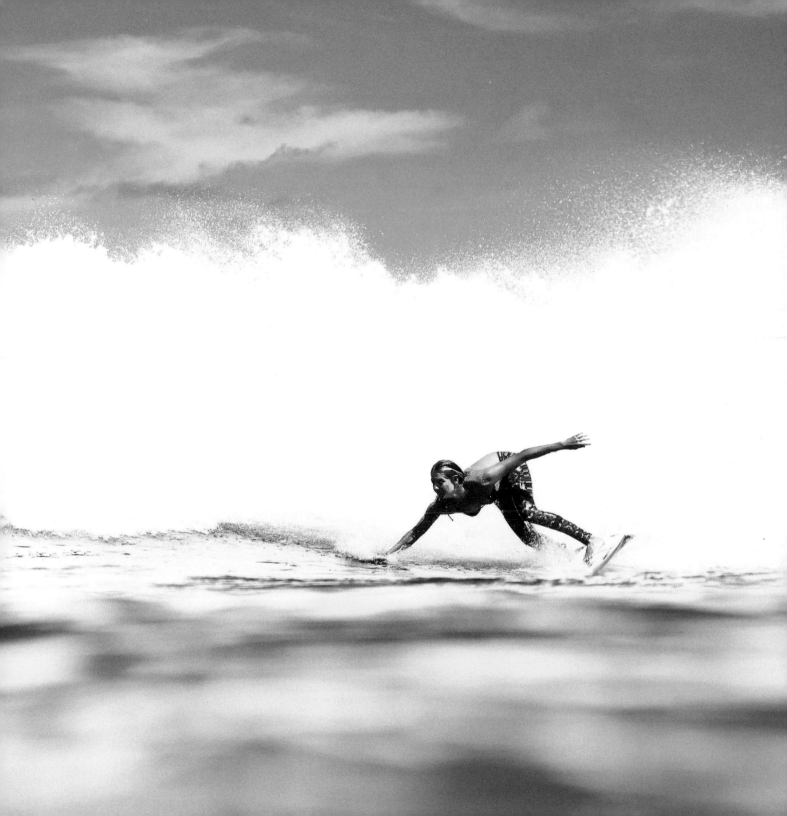

explosive power

Explosive leg power is vital in surfing – whether you're charging off the lip or simply popping up onto your board in crumbly waves. Plyometric training may be just what you need to get you into bombs that little bit earlier, or to boost your summer wave count.

What is plyometric training?

Plyometric training is a type of training designed to produce fast, powerful movements, which will improve the functions of the nervous system and enhance sports performance. Muscles are loaded and then contracted in rapid sequence, using the strength, elasticity and innervations of the muscle and surrounding tissues to jump higher, run faster, throw further or hit harder – depending on the training goal. As well as optimising explosive power, plyometric training will improve the ligaments, tendons and muscles of the legs, which can help in injury prevention.

Where do I start?

Before starting plyometric training it's advisable to do a basic warm up of at least 10 minutes. To get the best results you should aim to build each session up to at least 20 minutes, two to three times a week.

Are there any risks?

Like any impact exercise, plyometrics can increase the risk of injury if you don't follow some safety precautions. The tremendous force generated during these moves requires that you use them sparingly and with proper training.

The most important aspect of a safe and effective plyometric programme is developing a safe landing technique – landing softly on your toes and rolling to your heels. This helps dissipate the impact forces on your joints. The other key to a proper landing is to avoid any twisting or sideways motion at the knee.

Remember, using a soft surface and wearing correct shoes is very important.

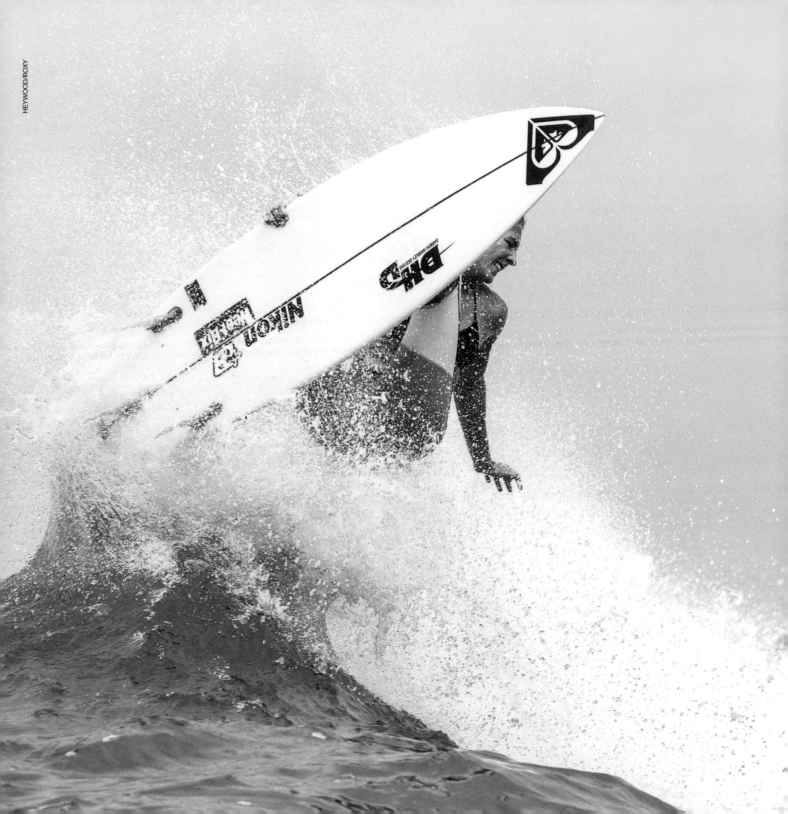

basic plyometric exercises

for boosting your explosive power

01. | Vertical Jumps

- Stand with your feet hip-width apart.
- Do a powerful jump upwards, taking 5 seconds rest between each jump.
  How many? Try at least 2 sets of 5 jumps

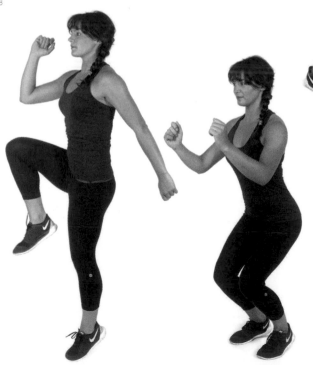

02. | Single Leg Vertical Jumps
(BEGINNERS)

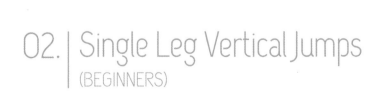

- Stand with legs at a 90-degree angle.
- With one big powerful movement, bring your knee up to your chest using your arms to aid the movement and add balance.

03. | Single Leg Jumps with Light Weights
(INTERMEDIATE)

- Complete the move in the same way as before, this time holding light weights to add resistance throughout the move

04. | Single Leg Jumps with Heavy Weights
(ADVANCED)

- Complete the move as before, only using a heavy weight.
(Do not attempt this if you are new to exercise or you have not yet developed to an intermediate level of strength).

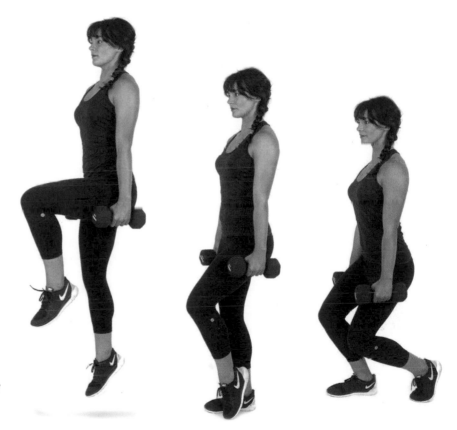

"Even very simple exercises such as a basic jump can be a great way to get extra leg strength."

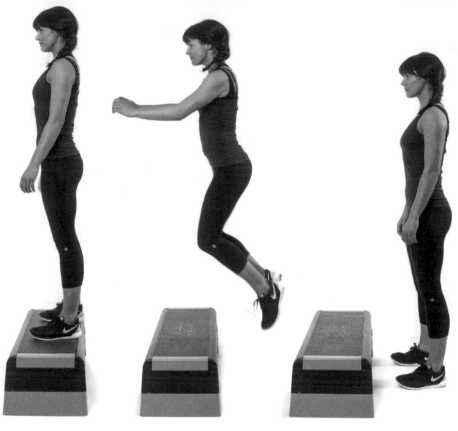

05. | Box Jumps

For this exercise you will need a box, or similar step that's about knee high. It's important to stay well focused during the movement to avoid injury.

- Start with feet slightly apart.
- Using your arms, jump up onto the box, then back down onto the floor again before repeating.

06. | Squat Thrusts

- Start the exercise in the press-up position, hands in line with your shoulders.
- Bring the knees forwards at speed, feet together, then quickly extend the legs back to the starting position.
- Repeat this 5 times before resting.

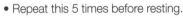
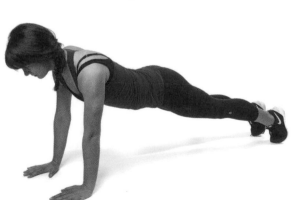
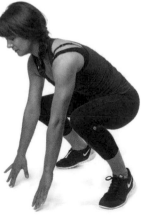
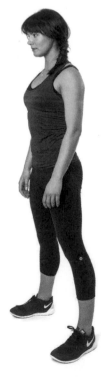

HEYWOOD/ROXY

Getting to
Your Feet

Squat Thrusts are a fantastic exercise
to practice getting to your feet and
popping up on your surfboard. As you
get stronger you may wish to increase
the reps. Try building up to 6x15 reps
and do this at least once or twice a
week to see improved results in your
pop ups. You can also add a jump up
at the each of each squat thrust.

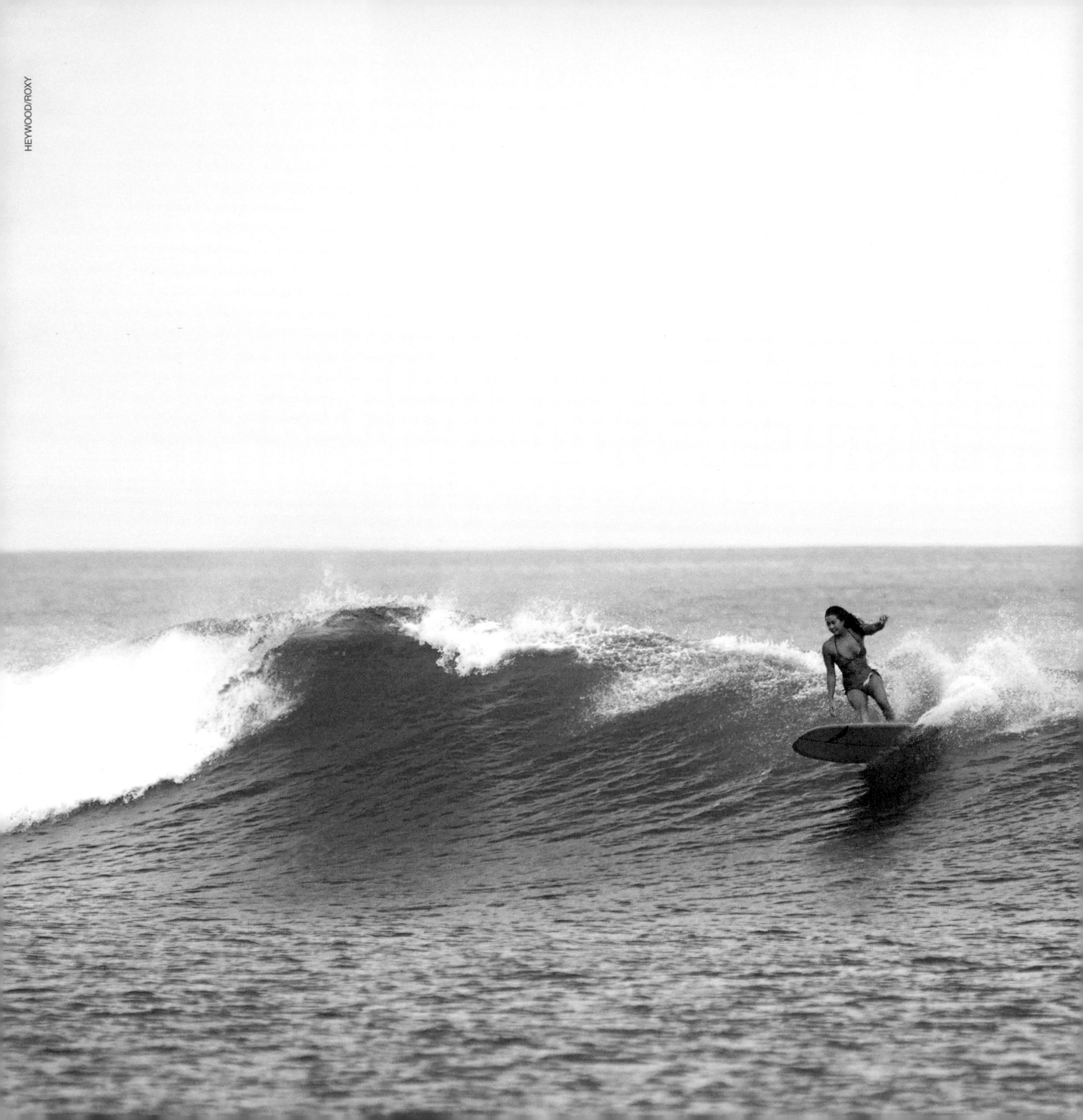

HEYWOOD/ROXY

TONE

STRENGTHEN

DETOX

dynamic
power exercises

PLYOMETRICS FOR EXPLOSIVE SURFING POWER
By using high-quality and multi-directional drills, explosive movement and response times can be improved. Speed and agility are undoubtably highly desirable qualities in all surfing movements. Basic plyometric training in your training programme will sharpen your surfing movements making them faster.

01. | Basic Step Up

- The basic step is simply a step up, but can be used at pace to improve aerobic fitness and leg strength.

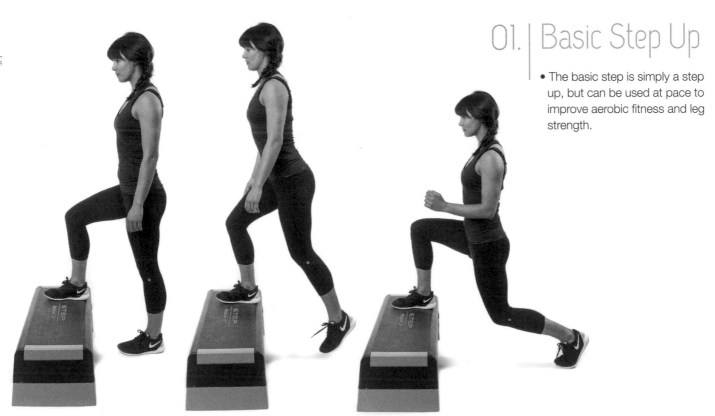

02. | Basic Step Up with Knee Raise

- Step up onto the box and as you do raise your knee extra high.
- Pause before stepping back down.
- Keep this going for 60 second intervals.

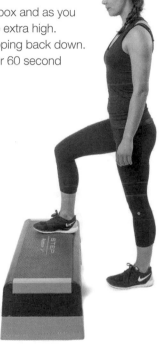
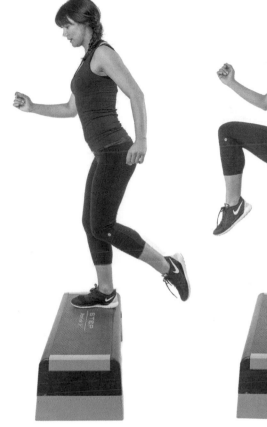
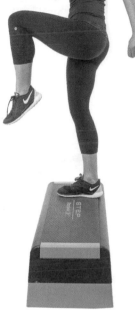

Increase Your Explosive Power using the Reebok Step

A very basic bit of training kit, the Reebok step is highly versatile. It can be used for a whole range of surf fitness training, from very simple exercises to advanced, aerobic and anaerobic training, strength training, and even core and balance training.

03. | Super Lunges with Weights

Leg strength is vital for surfing and sharper movements can be gained from an improvement in leg strength.

- Step forwards onto the box with weights hanging down by your sides.
- Lunge by lowering the trailing leg.
- Raise leg upwards, then back down to start position.

How many? Repeat 8 times and then change the start postition to work the opposite leg.

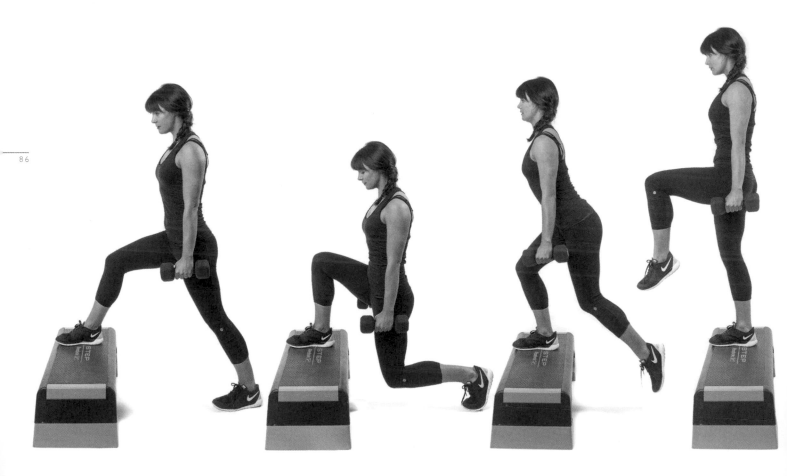

04. | Side Step at Pace

The side step is also a basic exercise, but can be used to boost aerobic and anaerobic fitness and improve coordination when done at speed.

• Start with feet on both sides of the step then, slowly to start with, step one foot up on the box followed by the other. As your co-ordination improves, increase speed.

• Work at intervals, improving your fitness by increasing your duration.

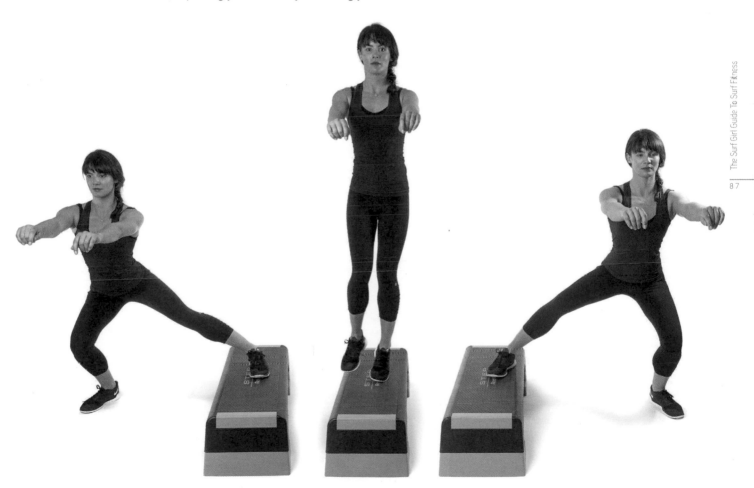

05. | Side Step with Weights (ALTERNATE ARMS)

- Again with a step, start the movement with one foot on the box.
- Step from side to side, swapping the weight from one hand to the other with the movement.

How many? Repeat 8-12 times.

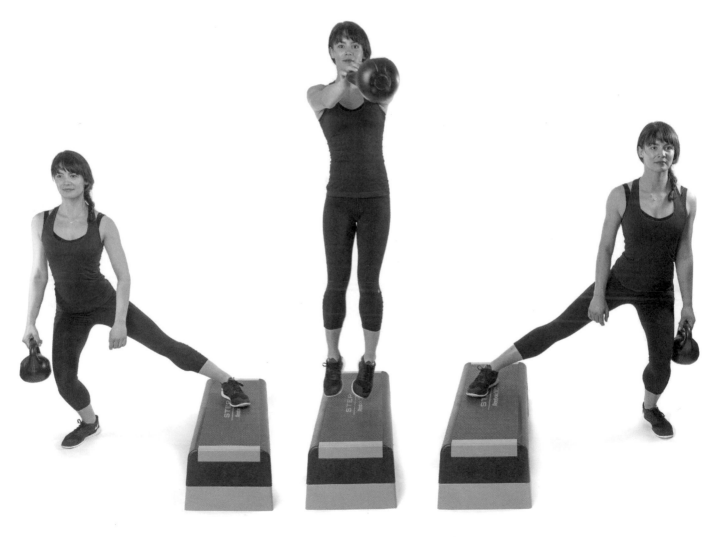

06. | Side Step with Weights

The side step is also a basic exercise, but can be used to boost aerobic and anaerobic fitness and improve coordination when done at speed.

- Start with feet on both sides of the step then, slowly to start with, step one foot up on the box followed by the other. As your co-ordination improves, increase speed.
- Work at intervals, improving your fitness by increasing your duration.

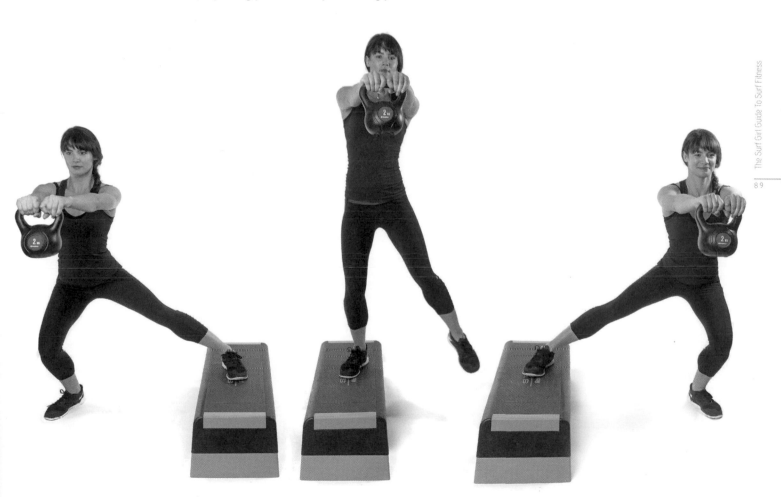

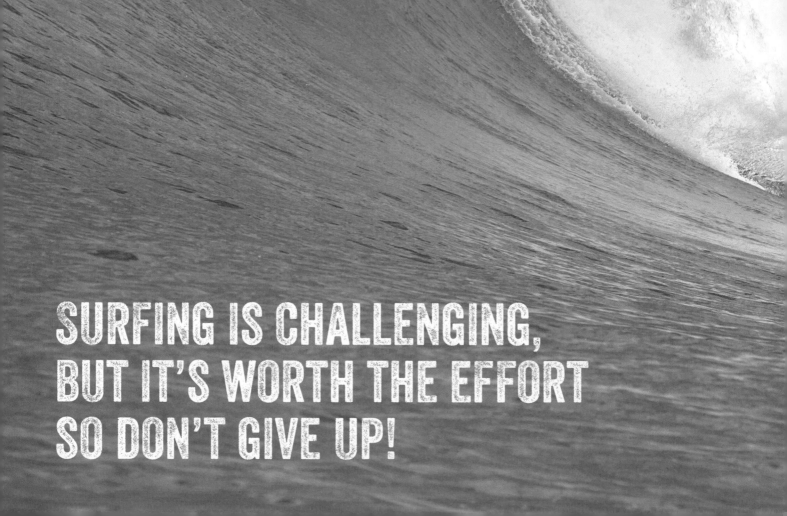

SURFING IS CHALLENGING,
BUT IT'S WORTH THE EFFORT
SO DON'T GIVE UP!

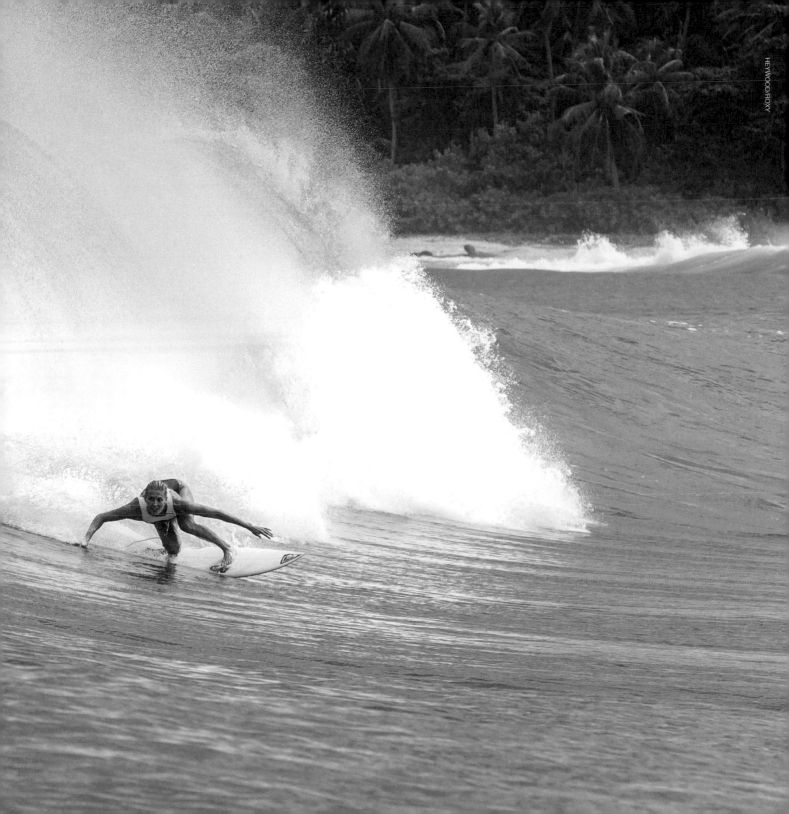

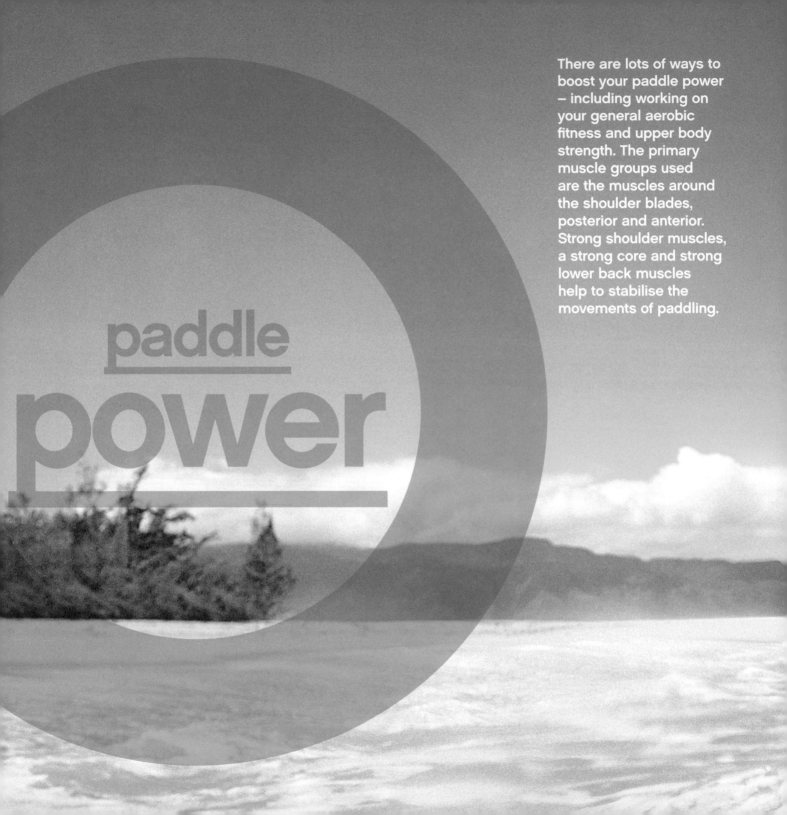

paddle power

There are lots of ways to boost your paddle power – including working on your general aerobic fitness and upper body strength. The primary muscle groups used are the muscles around the shoulder blades, posterior and anterior. Strong shoulder muscles, a strong core and strong lower back muscles help to stabilise the movements of paddling.

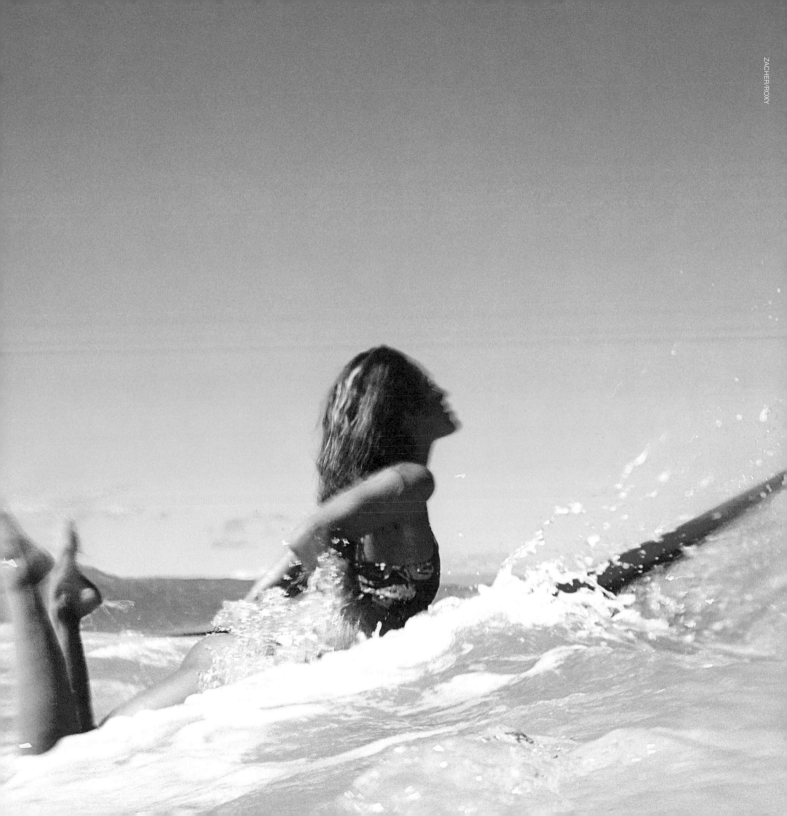

paddle power training

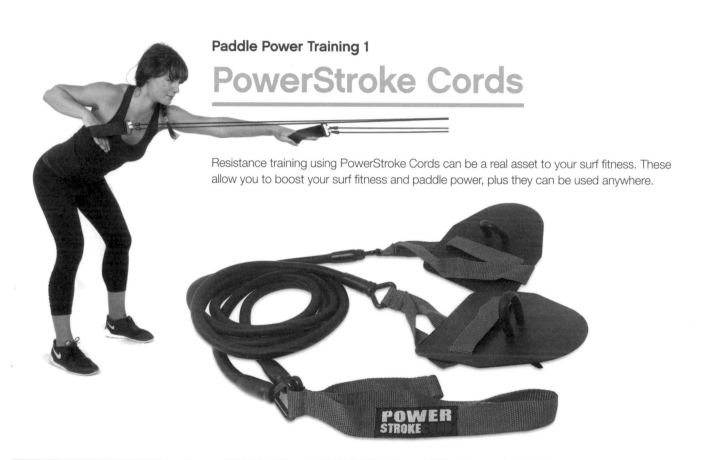

Paddle Power Training 1

PowerStroke Cords

Resistance training using PowerStroke Cords can be a real asset to your surf fitness. These allow you to boost your surf fitness and paddle power, plus they can be used anywhere.

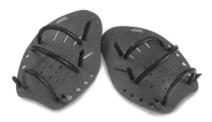

Paddle Power Training 2

Swim training with aids

Both recreational and elite swimmers use swim hand paddles, and these can be a real asset to the surfer looking for improvements in surfing paddle power. Hand paddles boost the muscles used in surfing paddle outs and wave catching. There are many different types and sizes – for more information go to Fit4swimming.com.

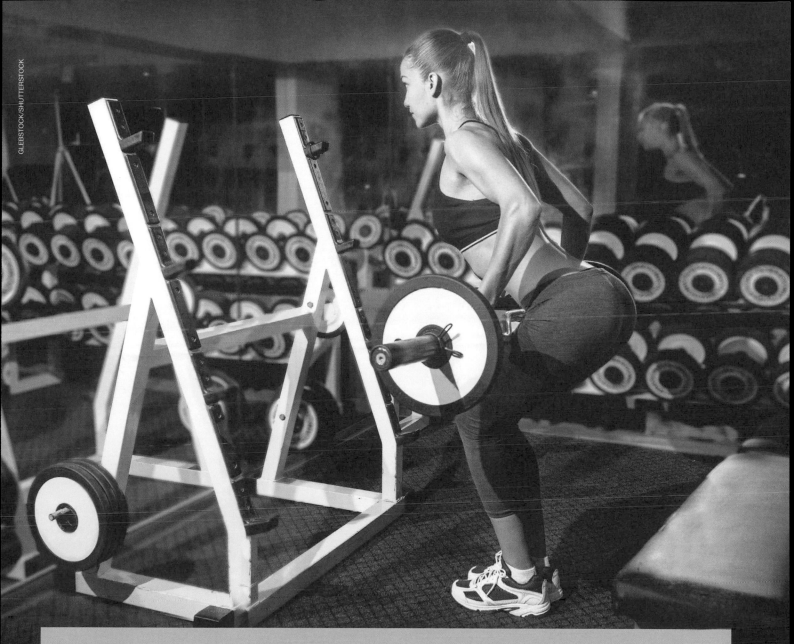
GLEBSTOCK/SHUTTERSTOCK

Paddle Power Training 3

High repetition resistance training

Using free weights to improve strength and endurance is also a great way to increase your paddle power. Isolating the muscle groups that are used during the paddle out or wave catching will see improvements, especially when used in conjunction with resistance cords.

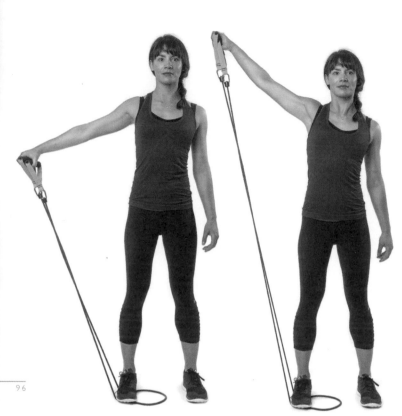

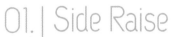

01. | Side Raise

- Place your PowerStroke Cords on the floor.
- Keeping in line with your body, slowly raise upwards.

How many? Repeat 8-10 times.

02. | Front Raise

- Start by standing on the cord.
- In line with your body, raise upwards.

How many? Repeat 8-10 times.

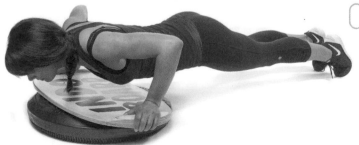

03. | Indo Deck Press-up

- Start in a press-up position, hands on the deck on a Gigante cushion.
- Lower down and hold.

How many? Repeat 8-10 times.

Boosting your paddle power is a must. The PowerStroke Cords can be used here to isolate the muscle groups used for paddling into that perfect wave. One of the most important muscle groups involved with paddling is the back of the arms – the muscle group known as the triceps.

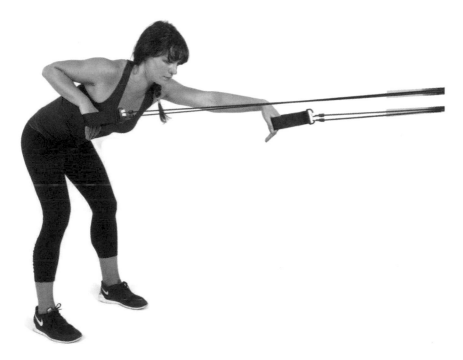

For sprint training try 10x20 seconds fast with 30 seconds rest after each 20 second sprint

Example PowerStroke Cords Workouts:

Beginner

- Do 5x60 seconds at a moderate pace with light breathing. Paddle slowly with smooth controlled movements. After each 60 seconds of paddle take 30 seconds rest.
- After 2 minutes of rest try 4x2 minutes of paddle taking 30 seconds rest.
- And finally try 3x3 minutes of paddle taking 45 seconds rest after each 3 minutes.
- Cool down with 10 minutes light stretching.

Intermediate

- Warm up with 5 minutes mobility exercises.
- 5x2 minutes light paddle with 30 seconds rest after each 2 minutes.
- Then do 4x3 minutes with 30 seconds rest after each 30 seconds.
- And finally try 1x5 minutes non-stop light paddle.
- Cool down with 10 minutes light stretching.

Advanced

- Warm up with 5 minutes mobility exercises.
- 10x2 minutes light paddle with 30 seconds rest after each 2 minutes.
- Then do 5x4 minutes at a strong to moderate pace with 60 seconds rest after each 4 minutes.
- Also try a 10 minute non-stop paddle.
- Cool down with 10 minutes light stretching.

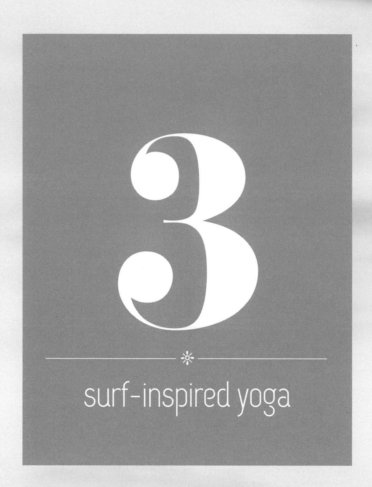

3

☀
---

surf-inspired yoga

IF YOU SURF AND YOU HAVEN'T TRIED INCORPORATING YOGA INTO YOUR TRAINING SCHEDULE, YOU'RE MISSING OUT. HERE WE LEARN HOW YOGA CAN HELP YOU FEEL GOOD ABOUT YOUR BODY AND BENEFIT YOUR SURFING.

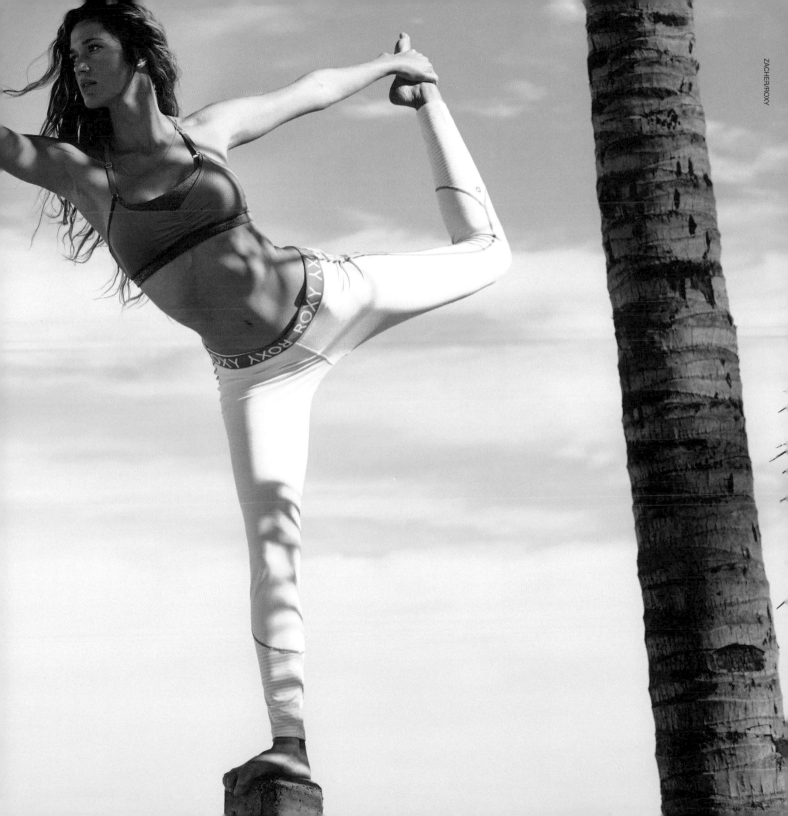

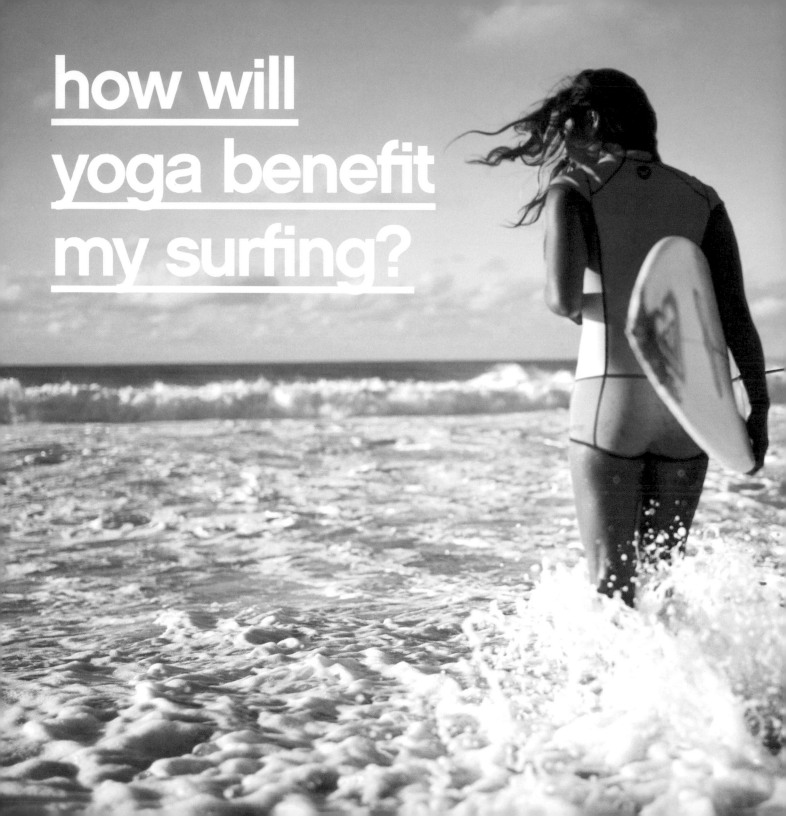

how will
yoga benefit
my surfing?

- Improved technique through fine-tuning the body.
- Improved stamina in the water.
- Better mental clarity and focus.
- Improved bone strength and flexibility.
- Better circulation, heart and lung health.
- Boost metabolism and detoxify the system.

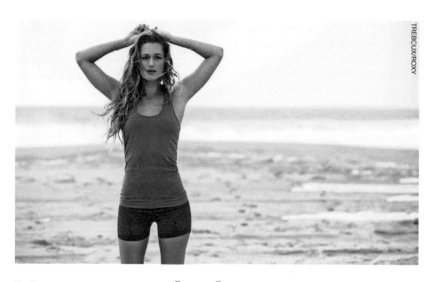

Yoga can help you maintain your fitness on many levels

A good range of motion will improve your turns and movement, helping to improve the flow of your body and surfing style through enhanced flexibility and limb awareness. Yoga will also help keep you in the water for longer by improving your strength and muscle efficiency through standing postures, arm balances and abdominal/core strengthening postures. Building up the strength in your legs will improve the power in your turns and resist 'jelly legs' syndrome on longer rides. Core strength will help to stabilise the body and improve balance, as well as help you to get to your feet quicker and more accurately. Upper-body strength is crucial to improving your surf stamina, and yoga can work on your arms, shoulders and lats, benefitting your paddle power.

Regular yoga practice can help to rebalance your body, mind and spirit, upping your positivity levels and generally improving your mental and physical functionality, creating a better balance to your surfing and to your life. The combination of yoga and a mindful approach to surfing could also help to control anxiety in the water when surfing bigger waves. Basically, committing yourself to just a few minutes of yoga each day could have a profound effect not only on your surf stamina, but also increase your self-esteem, mood and confidence, and your general well-being and quality of life.

Where Do I Start?

You don't have to be a yogi to enjoy yoga. Start by looking at individual postures that will help maintain physical fitness or improve your water time. For those interested in learning the deeper content of practice, starting with the fundamental principles of yoga is advised, which inevitably leads us to develop spiritual awareness.

To improve your surfing through yoga, stick to some simple rules: be kind, don't push your body beyond its limits, be patient and have gratitude for your body and for nature's playground, and open your eyes to the interconnection of all things through yoga practice.

Breathing

Pranayama, or breathing exercises, will improve lung health and capacity, making duck diving and 'hold downs' during bigger sets more comfortable. It can also help you to become more mindful and shift from a fragile state to a more calm state when a big swell is on its way. Pranayama dissolves negative thought by focusing the mind and improving bodily functions, particularly respiratory and digestive functions. It is also a great way to centre yourself in preparation for meditation, as it helps to burn off agitation, and to balance both hemispheres of the brain.

How do I do it?

Simple, conscious breathing is a form of Pranayama and is a brilliant way to start your day. You don't have to practice intense sequences of breath-work, instead be guided by your natural breath until it opens up in its own time. Then focus on breathing a little deeper, experiencing the physiological effects – the slowing of your heartbeat, the lifting and spreading of your ribcage, the stretching of the intercostal muscles and the lifting of your spine on inhalation and the retraction on exhalation.

Try this:

Focus on your natural breath and notice where the breath reaches – is there any tightness, are you restricted, are you breathing into just the chest or into the upper lobes of the lungs? Relax the belly and inhale slowly. Imagine the breath travelling down into your belly (try not to push your stomach out). As you exhale let go of tension from the shoulders and the whole body. Exhale away all tension as the navel gently retracts back towards the spine. Repeat several times.

Meditation

Meditation has profound health benefits. Working with visualisation can be a beautiful meditation when you're land-locked or during a flat spell. However, you do not have to work with visualisation or do any spiritual ritual to meditate: simply sitting comfortably, watching the breath with conscious breathing (see right), helps reduce stress and pressure on the body and mind.

Try this:

As you practise the breathing technique, notice any thoughts that arise. In the beginning there will be many. Watch the thoughts as they unfold, and then let them go. Be non-judgmental, with no attachment to the thoughts. Avoid building stories, see the thoughts and acknowledge them, and then just let them go.

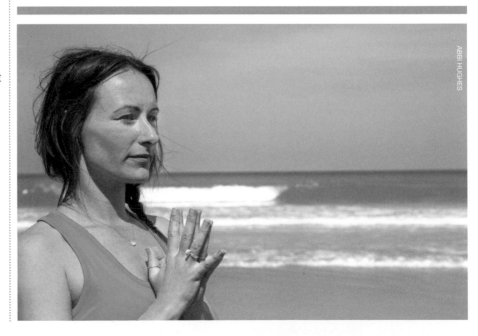

ABBI HUGHES

Visualisation

Visualisation can help reduce anxiety and improve performance. For a long time sports psychologists have used visualisation for athletes.

Try this surfing meditation before your next surf:

Sit comfortably on a chair and close your eyes. Relax your body, paying particular attention to any tension in your jaw, neck and shoulders. Let your hands relax into your lap, take a deep breath and sigh out all tension from the body. Now imagine you are sitting on your board out back: It's a beautiful day, there's no agenda, you are just experiencing this beautiful environment. Take in the light – are there any clouds or are you glowing in the sunrise or sunset? Imagine your environment and be creative. You might start to notice the swell, building to perfect, glassy-faced wave sets. Visualise your perfect wave and paddle into it. Feel the power of the wave lift your board and jump to your feet, stable, held by the wave, enjoying the best wave of your life.

Tip: If you struggle with anxiety in big waves then practice the visualisation as above, and as you see the wave beginning to form, notice your body's response: have you tightened up? Try relaxing the body and stepping back into the enjoyment of the experience… let go.

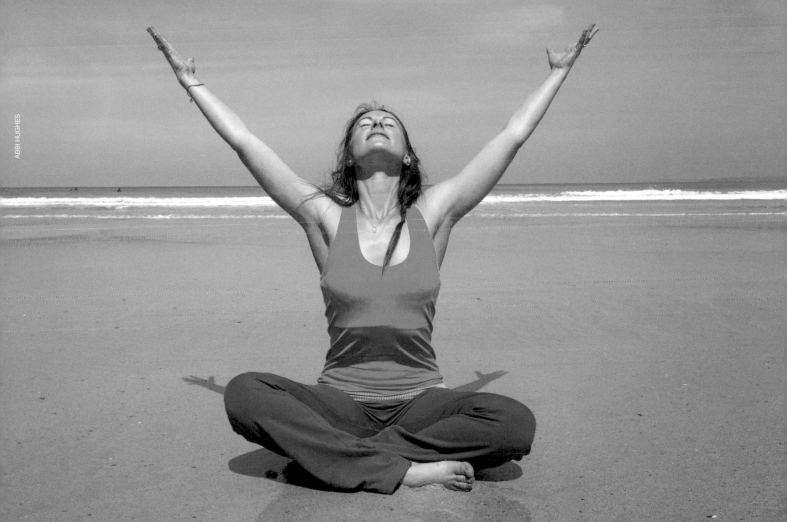

ABBI HUGHES

LOOK AROUND YOU,
EMPTY YOUR THOUGHTS AND BREATHE.

ENJOY THE LITTLE THINGS

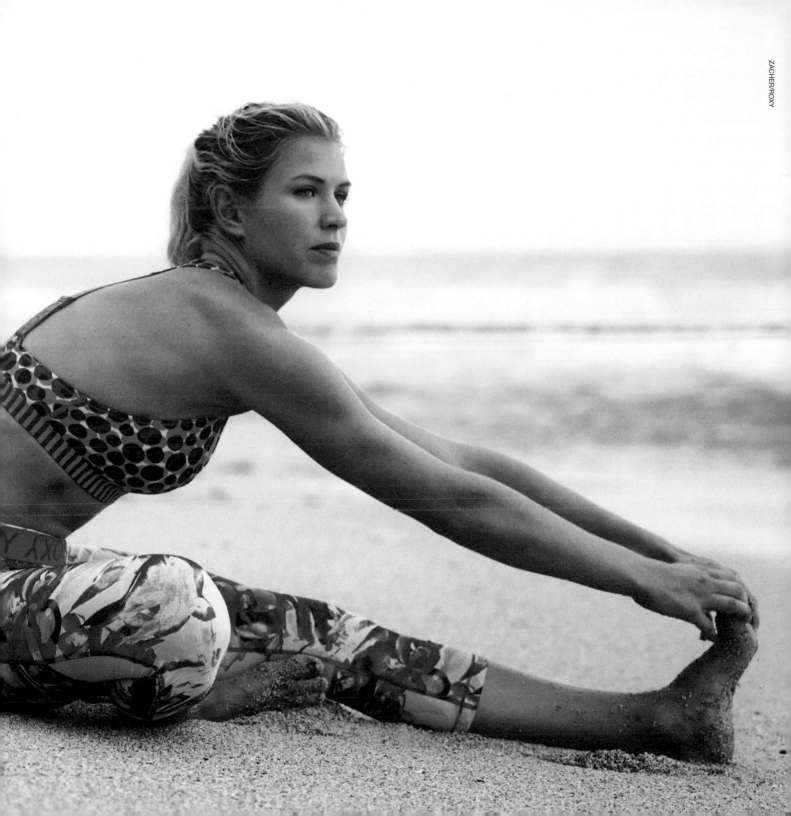

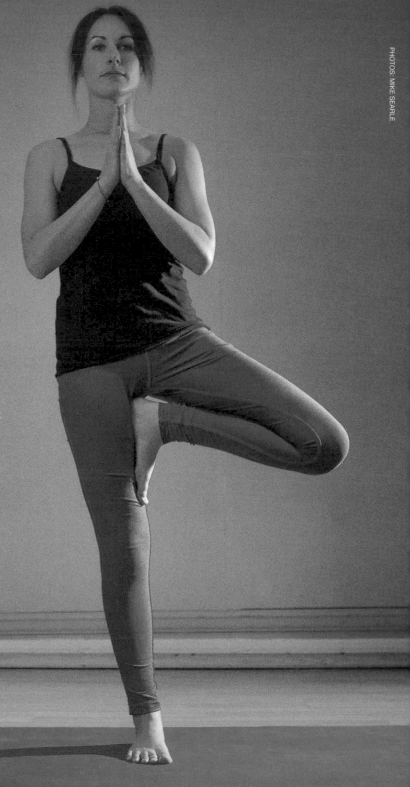

01 | Vrksasana
TREE POSE

Benefits: Strengthens the intrinsic muscles of the feet and ankles. The thighs, calves, ankles and spine get stronger, the groin and inner thighs are stretched, and chest and shoulder mobility is improved with prayer positioning of hands. Helps to relieve sciatica and improves your balance and mental focus both in and out of the water.

• Standing in Tadasana (feet together), engage the bandhas (pelvic floor and lower abdominals) and bring one foot up to the inner thigh.
• Take the hands to the hips briefly, to check the alignment of the hips and that the pelvis is balanced after lifting the leg. Press the palms together at the heart centre.
• Press the foot into the thigh and the thigh back into the foot, shifting the knee to the back of the room.
• Find balance through the continued contraction of the transverse abdominal (Uddiyana Bandha) and fix your gaze on a point ahead of you.
• Breathe fully but softly.
• To modify and intensify this posture, try reversing the prayer hands position behind the back (be sure to pull the front ribs in to soften and bring length into the lumbar spine and lower back).

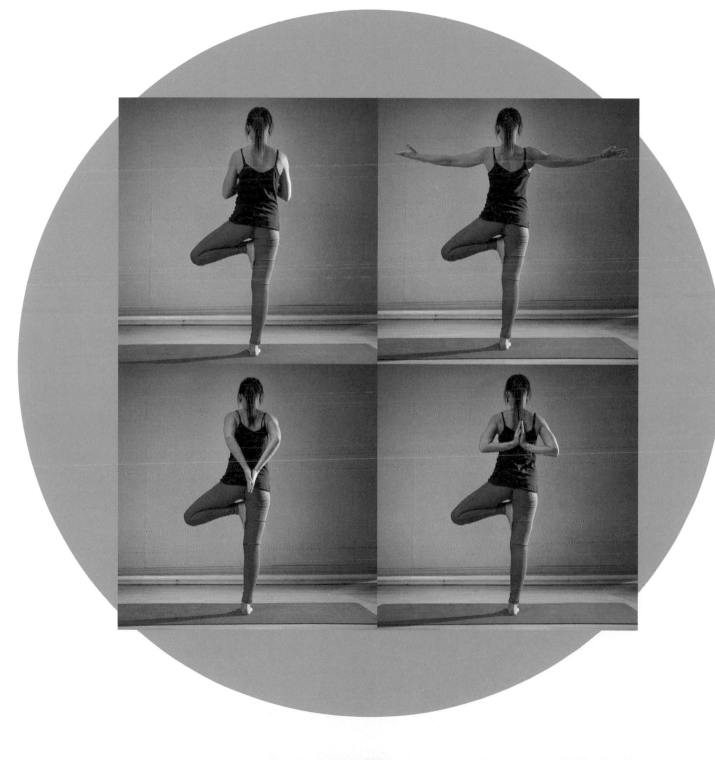

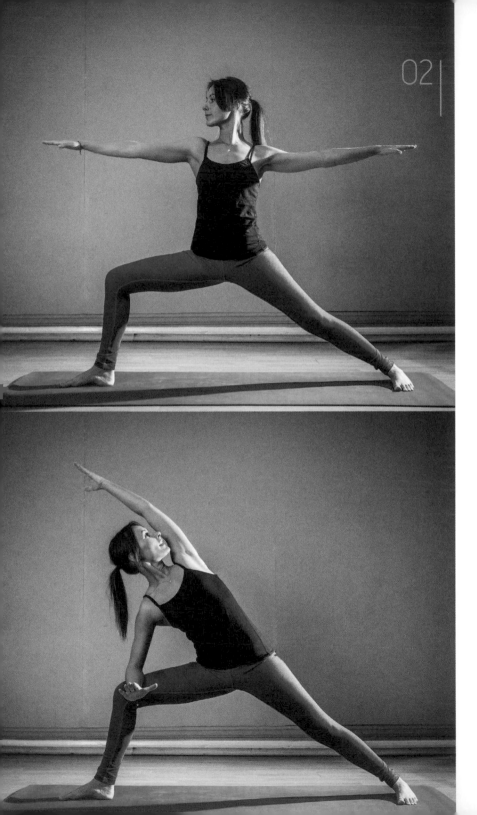

Virabhadrasana 2 into Parsvakonasana
WARRIOR 2 INTO EXTENDED SIDE ANGLE POSE

Benefits: Strengthens and stretches the legs and ankles, increasing power in your turns. Stretches the side body, chest, lungs, groin and shoulders. A grounding posture that also stimulates abdominal organs, and increases strength and stamina.

- From the front of your mat step one foot back.
- Kick the back heel out a couple of inches so the foot is angled, align the front leg in a 90-degree position, toes pointing towards the front of the mat (make sure the front heel cuts through the centre/arch of the back foot for correct alignment).
- Inhale, then as you exhale bend the front knee (keep an eye on your alignment), press the front knee out to align it above the ankle and keep the back leg strong.
- Press down through the little-toe side of your back foot and allow your tailbone to descend. Arms are extended out at shoulder level and the pelvis and chest stay square.
- Gaze over the front hand and breathe.
- Inhale to transition into Parsvakonasana, and as you exhale drop your front arm onto the front thigh, press down with the forearm to lift and roll the ribcage to the sky, and reach the back arm either to the sky or towards the front of your mat.
- In both postures work to drop the back of the pelvis and lift the pubis, drop down through the little-toe side of the back foot throughout, and use the back leg as an anchor.

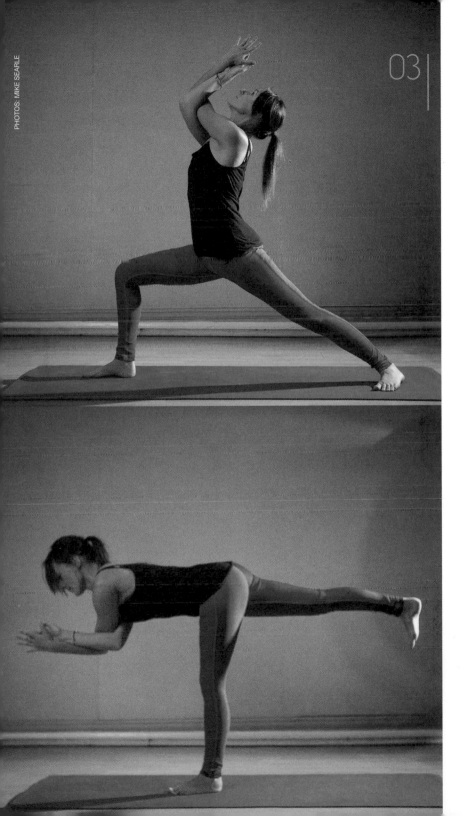

03 | Virabhadrasana 1 into Virabhadrasana 3
WARRIOR 1 INTO WARRIOR 3

Benefits: Stretches and opens the back, arms and shoulders ready for paddling. Strengthens the legs, core and the muscles of the back. Stretches and tones the thighs and calves, strengthen the ankles, and improves balance and mental focus.

- From the front of your mat step one foot back, making sure that the hips, chest and torso are still pointing towards the front of your mat.
- Pull the front thigh back to help align the pelvis and torso.
- Inhale the arms straight up to the sky, and as you exhale bend the front knee to take the front leg to a 90-degree angle. To protect your knee make sure that it stacks above the ankle and not past it.
- Maintain alignment by lifting the front of the pelvis and pulling the front ribs in.
- Create 'eagle arms' to challenge yourself in the pose: cross one arm on top of the other and hinge at the elbows, wrap the forearms and try to bring the palms together.
- Lift the elbows on an inhalation, and as you exhale pull the hands out from the face to intensify the release in the upper back. Gaze up to extend the spine.
- To transition into a balance, maintain the bind of the eagle arms and inhale, then as you exhale bring the chest forward and straighten the front, supporting leg. Allow the shift in your weight to counterbalance and transition you smoothly into the Warrior 3 variation.

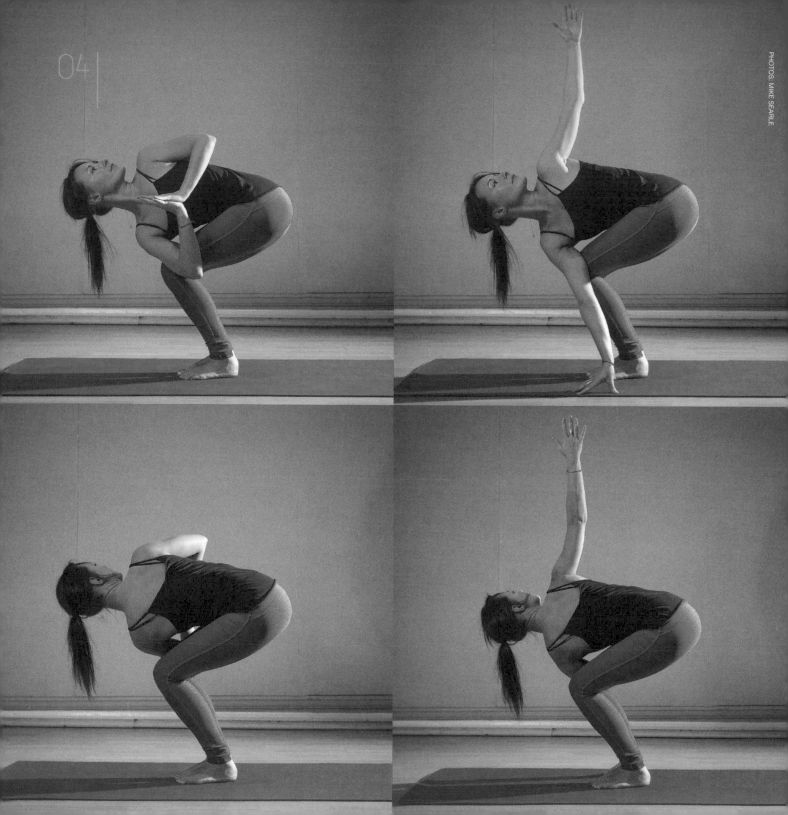

Utkatasana
CHAIR POSE

Benefits: Stimulating the liver, kidneys and spine. Strengthens the ankles and legs and stimulates the abdominal organs improving digestion. Twists are ideal for preparing for turns in the water.

- Come into Utkatasana by standing with your feet together, inhale the arms above the head and exhale the hips into a squat position.
- Draw your weight back into your heels and keep the knees together.
- Engage your core and lift the front of your pelvis up away from your thighs to create space in the front of the hip.
- Soften the front ribs, as if shifting the front ribs back into the body, this will ease lumbar spine compression, compliment this by lengthening the tail bone down.
- To modify into Parsva Utkatasana take a twist from your 'Chair pose' or squat position by inhaling and on your exhalation seal the hands together in prayer position at the centre of the chest as you twist to one side.
- Hook your underneath elbow to the outer thigh/knee, glance at the knees, check they are aligned to help keep the pelvis in the correct position, now bring the thumbs to a more central position in the chest to encourage the twist to deepen.
- Try taking one hand to the floor and extending the opposite arm up to the sky for a fun variation!
- Extend the ribs and spine forwards as you sink the hips deeper to intensify and gaze over the top shoulder for five full breaths.

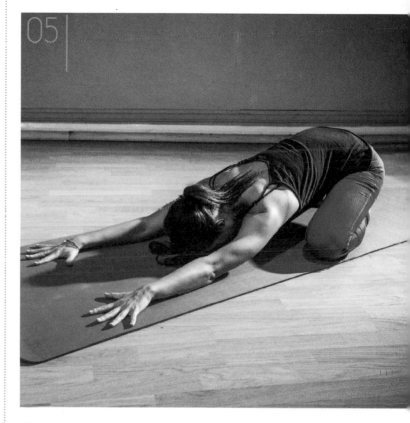

Balasana
CHILD'S POSE

Benefits: Stretches the spine, relieving backache and compression of the lumbar vertebrae (lower back) – making it ideal for after paddling sessions where the spine is in extension for long periods of time. Gently stretches the thighs, hips and ankles, and calms the mind, relieving stress and fatigue.

- From kneeling, reach the hands forward and sink the hips back to the heels, resting the forehead on the ground.
- As you take some deep breaths, feel the belly expand into the inner thighs.
- Continue to creep the hands forward with each inhalation and sink the hips back and down as you exhale.
- To stretch the inner thighs more, separate the knees wider apart.

PHOTOS: MIKE SEARLE

06 | Camatkarasana
WILD THING POSE

Benefits: This is an energising posture which stimulates the front body, stretches the hip flexors, abdomen, chest and shoulders. This posture will also encourage strength in the shoulder and upper back region. This is a strong pose! Warm up the back, shoulders and legs before attempting this posture, take it slowly, do not push too hard and practice to your limits, avoid if you have shoulder injury, rotator cuff issues or carpal tunnel syndrome.

- Start in Downward Facing Dog pose.
- Engage the bandhas, core, throughout.
- Elevate your right leg to the sky, bend your knee and kick the heal over towards the left side of your mat opening up the hip.
- After several breaths here, inhale and on the next out breath lift your right hand off the mat and allow your right leg to drop back.
- Stay up on the toes of your right leg, heel lifted and reach your right arm either up to the sky or if you feel stable in the pose reach the hand back.
- On each inhale lift the hips and curl back to encourage the benefits of opening the front body in this pose.

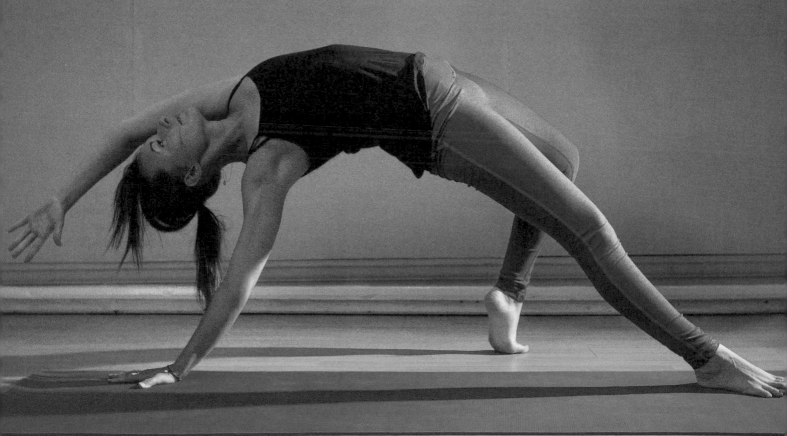

07 | Adho Mukha Svanasana
DOWNWARD-FACING DOG

Benefits: **Downward Dog stretches the entire length of the back body, soothes the mind and helps to relieve stress. It also strengthens the arms, shoulders and legs, improves digestion and reduces fatigue. The twisting variation stimulates the abdominal organs and improves digestion, as well as stretching the hip flexors and strengthening the legs.**

- From Child's pose, curl the toes under and lift the hips up and back to create an upside down 'V' shape with the body. To intensify the stretch, press the thighbones to the back of the room and descend the heels down towards the ground.
- Ground through the base of the index finger and thumb, and squeeze the forearms towards one another, lifting the shoulder away from the ears and rolling the upper arms outward to spread into the upper back.
- Engage the bandhas (lower abdomen and pelvic floor) throughout.
- Avoid locking the knees, instead bend the knees a little, pull up through your thighs and then on an exhale straighten the legs – this will avoid hyperextension through the backs of the knees (the same applies to working the muscles in the arms to protect and support the elbow joints).

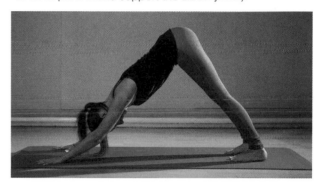

08 | Bakasana into Astavakrasana
CROW POSE INTO EIGHT-LIMBED POSE

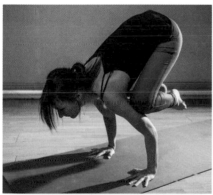

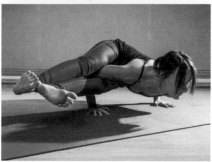

Benefits: **Improves balance and arm/wrist strength – ideal for pop-ups! Stretches the upper back and strengthens, tones and stimulates the abdominal muscles. In balancing postures the mind is focused, improving mental clarity.**

- Come down to the floor with your knees together and perch on your toes.
- Now separate your knees wide apart and reach your arms forward, planting the hands down shoulder distance apart and lifting the hips.
- As you gaze forward transfer the weight into the hands, lifting the knees as high up into the armpit as possible.
- PLAY! Try taking one foot off the ground then the other (keep looking ahead to avoid falling forwards). Once you have lift-off, work to straighten the arms.
- To transition into Astravakasana, make sure you are warmed up well and take it easy if you are new to this transition.
- From Bakasana, send your left leg through the arms, bend at the elbows and dip your chest closer to the ground as you straighten out the right (top) leg and cross the ankles.
- Look ahead and breathe!

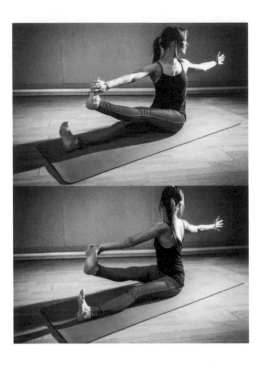

09 | Seated Twist

Benefits: Manipulates the abdominal organs, including the liver and kidneys. Stretches the shoulders, hamstrings and calves, relieves back tension, opens the chest and strengthens and stretches the spine.

- Sitting in a 90-degree position with the legs out straight, lengthen the spine and engage the bandhas (abdominals).
- Bend one knee and reach the opposite hand across the midline of the body to catch the outer foot of the opposite leg. If your hamstrings are tight and you cannot straighten the leg, use a belt instead and loop it around the foot.
- Now begin to twist from the navel, taking the opposite arm towards the back of the room. If you struggle to sit up tall and feel a strain in your back, have a go at sitting on the edge of a folded blanket.
- Take 5 deep breaths.

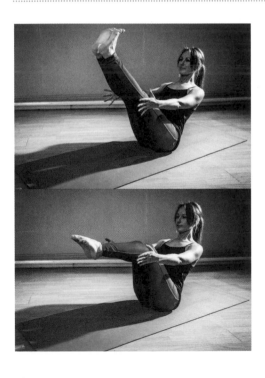

10 | Navasana
BOAT POSE

Benefits: Strengthens the core improving strength, stamina and balance in the water. Strengthens hip flexors and spine, and improves digestion.

- Sit on the floor with your knees bent and feet together in front of you.
- Pull your belly in, lift the chest and lean back slightly to elevate the legs.
- Take the legs to a 90-degree angle. If that feels okay on your back, extend both of your arms forward to challenge your core and your balance.
- Work to lift the knees towards the chest and the chest towards the knees.
- Maintain bandhas and an even, flowing breath.
- To intensify and progress the pose, straighten the legs.

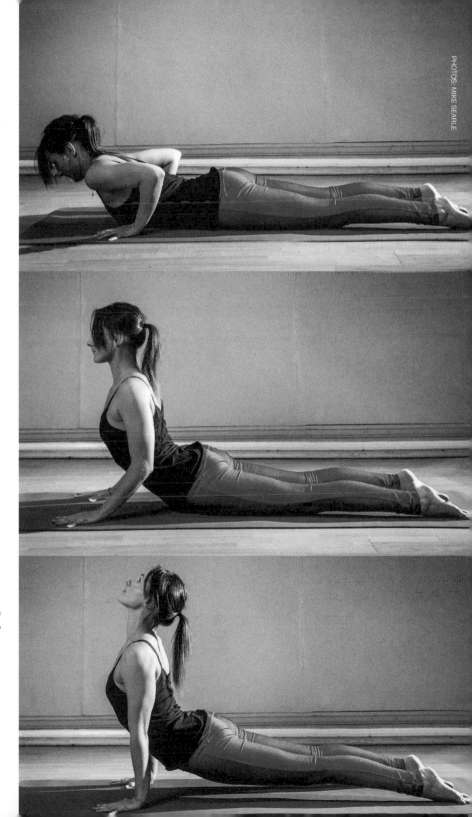

11 | Bhujangasana into Urdhva Mukha Svanasana
COBRA POSE INTO UPWARD-FACING DOG

Benefits: This pose is a great for surfing posture – it strengthens the spine and prepares the back for extension in paddling, while stretching the chest, lungs and shoulders. It also stimulates the abdomen, improves respiratoration, helps relieve fatigue and soothes sciatica.

- Lie on the stomach with bandhas (abdominals) engaged.
- Roll the inner thighs up and press through the tops of the feet, then lift the pubic bone up towards the navel as the tailbone descends between the heels.
- Roll the shoulders and inhale the chest off the ground (avoid compressing the lower back), squeeze the elbows in and make sure that you can wiggle your fingers so you're not over-working the arms.
- As you exhale, bring the chest forwards and down.
- Repeat 5-6 times.
- To transition into Upward Dog, repeat the adjustments of the lower half of the body and drag the hands back to waist level.
- Press down strongly through the hands and feet as you straighten the arms. The hips and knees should float up off the ground. Be here for 3-5 slow, steady breaths.

Benefits Stretches the entire front of the body – throat, chest, abdomen, thighs and ankles. Stretches the deep hip flexors and strengthens back muscles.

- Kneel on your mat with knees hip-distance apart and take the hands onto the hips.
- Drop your tail and lift the front of the pelvis up.
- Inhale and lift the rib cage to the sky, then exhale and reach the hands back to catch the heels. Press the fingers into the heels to encourage the lifting action of the chest and ribs.
- Maintain abdominal contraction throughout and take 5 breaths.

13 | Supine Twist

Benefits: Manipulates the abdominal organs, including the liver and kidneys. Stretches the shoulders, chest, hamstrings, hip and calves, relieves back tension, opens the chest and strengthens and stretches the spine.

- Lying in supine position on your back, bring the right knee across the midline of the body to the opposite side of the mat.
- As you roll the knee across, skip the hips to the right to keep the alignment of the pose and gaze over the right shoulder. The left hand supports the pose by resting on the outer right thigh.
- Press the right shoulder blade down towards the ground and take 5-8 breaths each side.

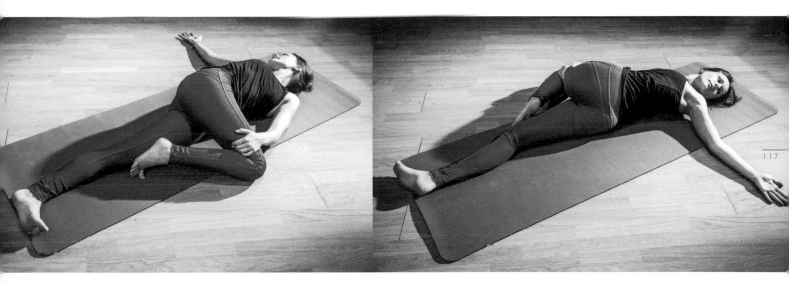

14 | Savasana
RELAXATION

- Lie on your back with your feet hip-width apart, arms by your sides and palms facing upwards.
- Drape a blanket over yourself and take 3-5 deep breaths to mark the end of your practice, quiet the mind and focus on releasing tension on each of your out breaths (sighing out the breath is a very useful technique).
- Then rest back into your natural breathing pattern. Stay here for 10-20 minutes. If the mind wanders gently bring it back to your breath, let thoughts come and then let them go, enjoying the tranquillity and quiet spaces that sit between your thoughts.

We're in awe of Stephanie Gilmore's endless optimism, passion for competition and indomitable spirit. With more World Titles than any other contender on the current women's tour combined, Steph continues to raise the bar of women's surfing with her powerful but fluid style on a board. She's an inspiration!

DREAM BIG
AND DARE TO FAIL

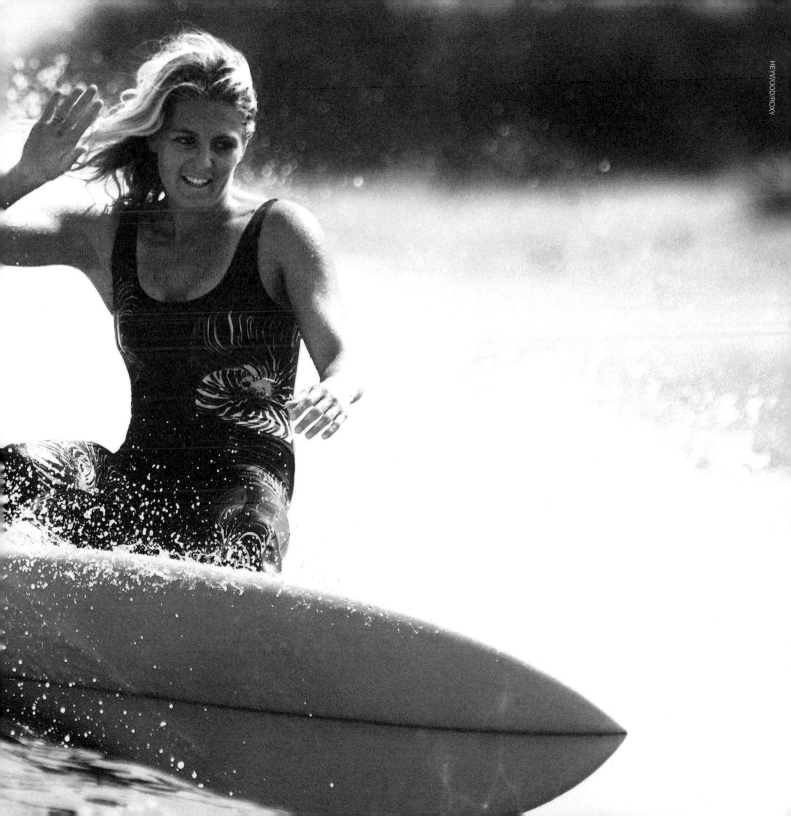

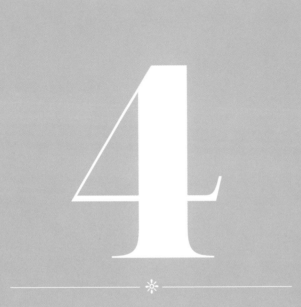

4

*

outdoor workout

FITNESS ISN'T ALL ABOUT GOING TO THE GYM; FEEL THE SAND BETWEEN YOUR TOES
AND THE SALTWATER IN YOUR HAIR WHEN YOU TRY THESE ALTERNATIVE FITNESS
ROUTINES AT THE BEACH. THE GREAT OUTDOORS IS AN AMAZING PLAYGROUND
WHERE YOU CAN GET FIT FOR FREE

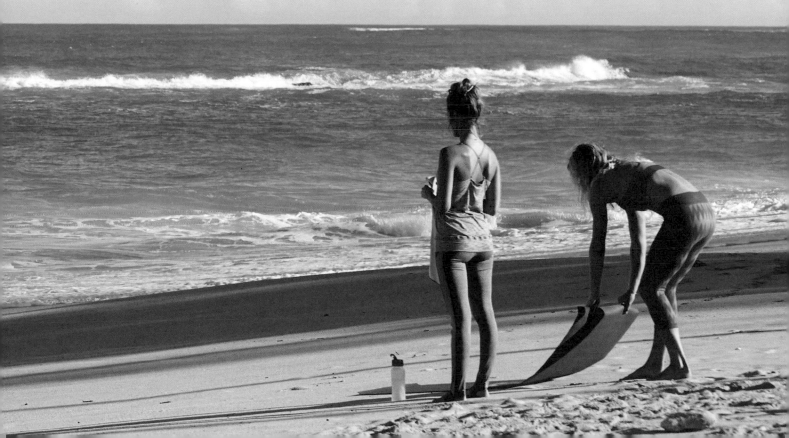

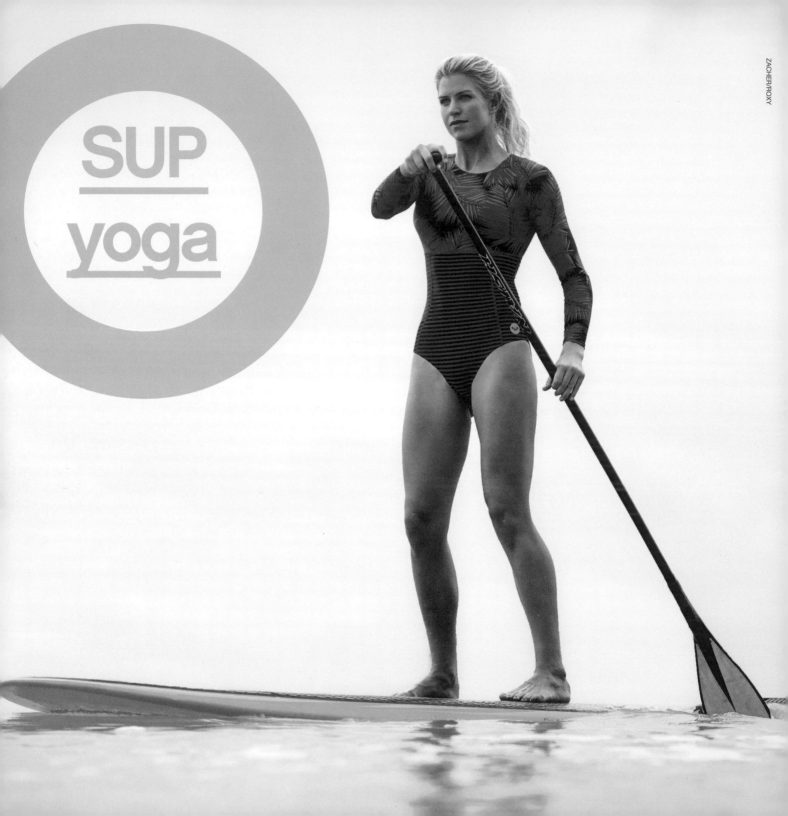

SUP
yoga

An avid surfer, yoga instructor and SUP enthusiast, Nat Fox has discovered the pure joy of SUP yoga.

"To be honest, when I first heard about SUP yoga I thought it was a bit of a gimmick – another fitness trend combining two different sports and techniques. Then I was asked to teach a class, and was hooked.

"The ocean has always felt like my spiritual home and I'm sure many surf girls feel the same: It's where my mind becomes clear, I feel connected to nature and everything is put into perspective. Yoga also has the power to bring me the same clarity and peace. So why not combine the two and transfer what I do on my yoga mat to a surface afloat in the sea? Stepping onto my SUP as if it was my yoga mat, it didn't feel gimmicky at all. Outdoors is my favourite place to do yoga, and this gave me the chance to practice yoga in my favourite environment – the ocean.

However, SUP yoga is also challenging. Sun salutations on a SUP take stability, balance and focus. Wobbles can turn into splashes and it's imperative to remain completely focused. While some yoga postures such as 'pigeon' and 'downward dog' are easy to transfer to a board, some inversions, standing postures and balances take some tweaking. Eventually I designed a routine that slowly worked towards a standing sun salutation, incorporating core-strengthening asanas, deeper stretches, a few playful balances and finishing with savasana – the ultimate relaxation posture.

"You never quite know where your surfing journey will take you. Once I dreamt I'd be surfing Pipeline, but now I approach surfing with an intention of connection – with nature and with my inner self. SUP yoga is a substitute when conditions don't allow for wave riding; it's a way that I can feel connected to the ocean, develop my awareness and balance, and exist in serene place and frame of mind.

"Don't take my word for its benefits – SUP yoga is definitely not gimmicky and you need to get out there for yourself try it for yourself!"

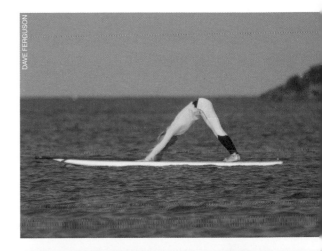

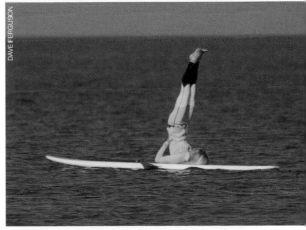

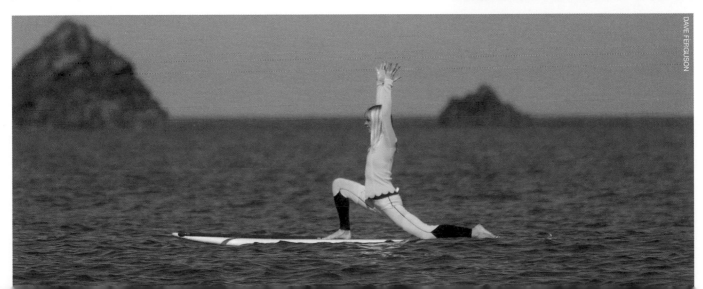

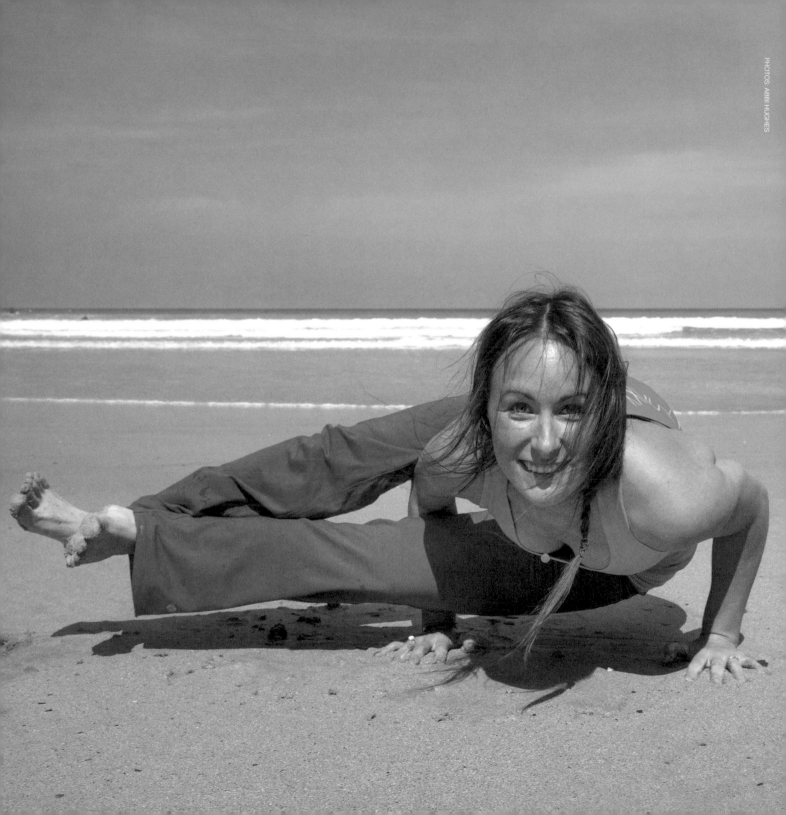

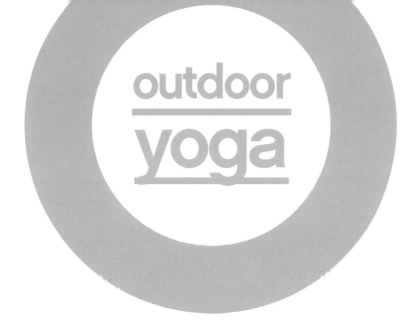

outdoor yoga

Yoga teacher Aimee Stapleford extols the joys of outdoor yoga.

"On those days when there's not a ripple in sight, beat the lull by getting out to play in nature. Taking your yoga outdoors will inspire your practice, call on all your senses and inject passion and positivity into your day. Getting up early to practice yoga can put a skip in your step: It increases self-esteem, mood, confidence and your general quality of life.

"The breath-work (known as Pranayama) combined with the physical movement of your body, boosts clarity and energises you. Yoga can help strengthen a positive mental attitude in and out of the water, and allows you take time out to reconnect with yourself.

"With regular yoga practice we soon realise why we commit to 6am alarm nudges and blurry-eyed sun salutations. Through yoga we really get to know ourselves, to reflect on what's real and what matters, instead of allowing the erratic mind to cloud our perceptions with its bombardment of cognitive – often negative, self-analytical – thoughts.

"Combine this mindfulness with the physiological bodily response of a boost to your metabolism and oxygenated blood pumping around the body, and a natural high is born! So get outside and stretch yourself. Outdoor yoga will lift your energy levels and your mind state, leaving you centred, blissed out and ready to enter back into your fast-paced life with a more humble and authentic perspective."

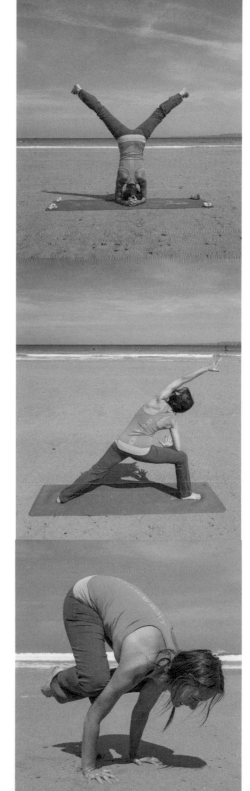

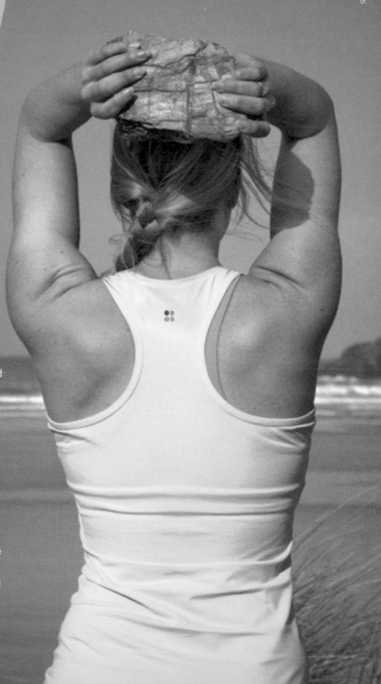

outdoor
gym

Head to the ultimate eco-gym: Fitness instructor Nathalie Frankson shows you how to use the beach as the ultimate place to workout.

"Shake off any inhibitions about exercising outside. Nothing rivals working out on the beach and it's the perfect antidote to time spent indoors. Jogging along the shoreline, immersed in the sounds and textures of the natural environment, will awaken your senses and give you a sense of freedom and adventure.

"Your body has to work much harder when you are on the sand – the uneven terrain both cushions and challenges your body, making you use many more stabilising and supporting muscles than you would in the gym, causing you to burn more calories and get fitter and stronger quicker."

Make an effort to leave your earphones behind and take a break from modern gadgets. While the light and landscape exercise your long-range vision after hours spent on the computer, some people believe that if you exercise barefoot on the beach you somehow earth the energy absorbed from technology!

When you look at the beach as your gym, it has everything you need to help work your body in different ways – whatever your fitness level and ability. There isn't even any need for weights as you can improvise with rocks and use your own body weight. The beach is the ultimate eco-gym.

To get you started, use this spring workout to get you in the mood and prepare you for your summer adventures:

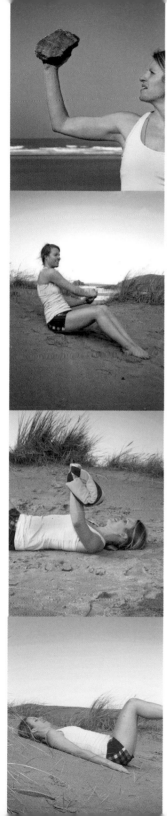

Beach Energiser

Simple running drills in the sand will strengthen, tone and energise you

1. **Steps:** The dunes act as a natural step machine. Choose your dune (make sure you aren't in a protected environment), run to the top, take a few breaths and walk down. Repeat five times.
2. **Sprints:** Draw your initial in the sand, then walk 50 paces and draw your initial in the sand again. Sprint between your markers up to ten times. Increase the intensity of your sprints by adding a set of knee lifts, squats and tuck jumps at either end.

Tone Up

Toning your upper body on the beach is simple. Work your pectoral (breast-supporting) muscles and tone your arms and shoulders with these exercises.

3. **Push ups:** Start off on your knees (you can progress to doing full press-ups on your toes), and keeping your abdominal muscles engaged, bring your hands just wider than shoulder-width apart and lower your chest to the ground. Perform 8 repetitions.

    Now bring your hands narrower and lower, towards your ribs, and do 4 narrow surfers' push-ups, as if you were going to pop-up on your board.

    Work even more muscles in your chest and core by performing your press-ups facing downward on a slight slope.
4. **Shoulder press and tricep extensions:** Grab a rock – choose a weight that feels challenging by 10-12 repetitions – and sit on the sand. Holding it in one hand, start off with your arm at 90 degrees and push the rock straight up. Perform 10-12 repetitions with each arm, then hold it in two hands above your head and lower it between your shoulder blades for 8 triceps extensions.

Surfside Abs

Why tone your abdominals inside when you can enjoy a sea view with every sit-up

5. **Crunches:** Sit on a slight slope and lay back in the sand. Bring your hands to your temples and do 10 abdominal crunches.
6. **Russian twists:** Stay sitting, but grab hold of the rock you were using for your shoulders and sit back 45 degrees. Hold the rock to the centre, twist through your torso to bring the rock towards the sand on your right, and then your left, for 16 repetitions.
7. **Leg extensions:** Lay back down on the sand, melting your body into the ground. Lift your legs up 90 degrees and carefully extend your right leg away and then your left, alternating up to 16 repetitions.

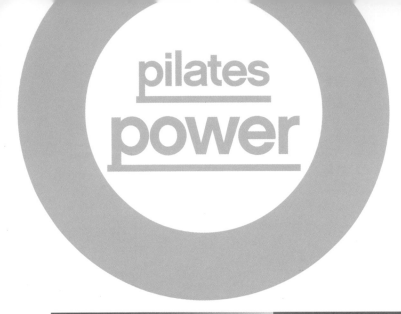

pilates power

Incorporating Pilates into your daily exercises can really help your surfing. Katie Watson, a physiotherapist and Pilates instructor at Flow Physio, shares a few core moves with us.

"Surfing puts all sorts of different demands on your body, and so surf fitness and improvement requires a varied approach, especially when it's difficult to get in the water regularly," explains Katie. "Encouraging core strength, control and flexibility, Pilates works well alongside surf fitness and will help you make the most of your time in the water. Try exercises such as the plank, press-ups, roll-downs, spine twists and the cobra, focussing on precision, control and quality of movement. Don't rush; take your time and enjoy learning what your body can do."

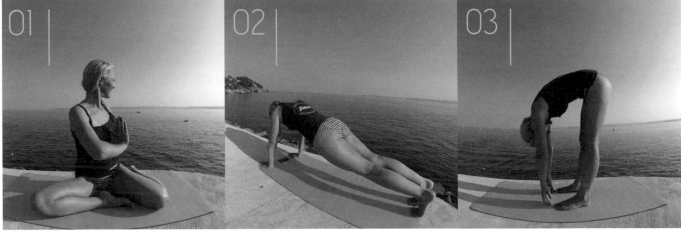

01 | SPINE TWIST

Placing your weight evenly between your sitting bones, and as you breathe out, rotate round. This is a great one to do before and after surfing.

02 | LEG PULL PREP

Keep your posture neutral and your shoulders and arms relaxed. You can also add a few press-ups in to make it harder – but always maintain a neutral posture. This is a great exercise to challenge the endurance of the whole body.

03 | ROLL DOWN

The surfer's staple exercise. Imagine you're unpeeling your back from the wall, vertebra by vertebra. Slowly lengthen towards the floor as you breathe out, then peel back up. Repeat and enjoy.

The powerhouse is the centre of the body and if strengthened, it offers a solid foundation for any movement. This power engine is a muscular network which provides control over the body and comprises all the front, lateral and back muscles found between the upper inner thighs and arm pits. – *Joseph Pilates*

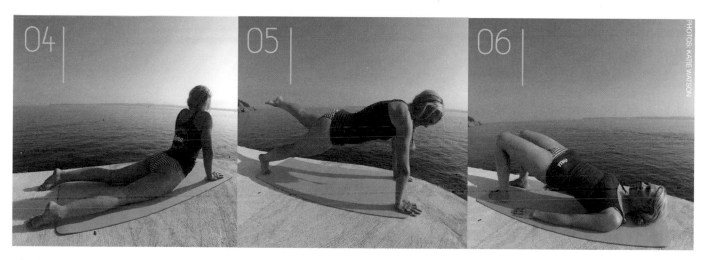

COBRA STRETCH

Facing the floor with your hips on the ground, breathe out and lengthen your spine upwards, extending across your collarbone and with your shoulders relaxed. You can also practice this without using your arms, to build the endurance of your back muscles for paddling.

LEG PULL PRONE

One step further on from the leg pull prep. Lengthen one leg away, keeping your pelvis neutral and your weight even. Keep your centre engaged to help control the movement.

SHOULDER BRIDGE

Slowly unpeel your spine from the mat, vertebra by vertebra, to bring yourself into a ski slope position. Keep your ribs relaxed into your abdomen – this helps isolate the movement of different parts of your spine. You can make it harder by extending one leg away, keeping your hips steady and your shoulders relaxed.

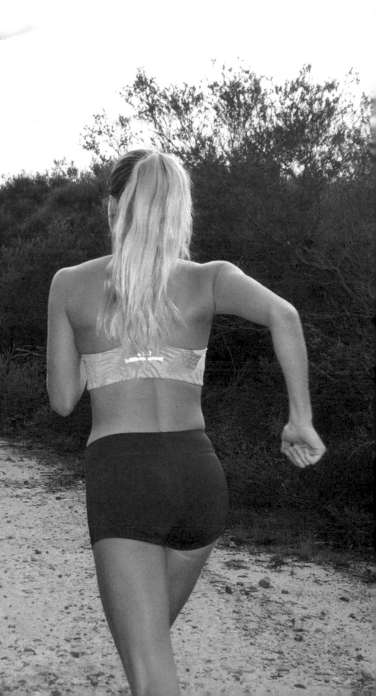

up and running

Surfer and triathlete Hayley Shaw McGuinness shows us how running can benefit your surf fitness.

"Running, you either love it or hate it. But even if you hate it, the great news is that you can learn to love it. Whatever you're running ability or goal – a 5km fun run, a 10km effort or a marathon – running is one of the most effective and accessible workouts you can do. It's free, offers a huge boost to your body, fitness and overall health, and it also comes with a giant bliss hit that makes it totally addictive."

How will running benefit my surfing?

Any aerobic training will have a positive effect on your overall fitness, which will improve your surfing performance. Running helps build strong bones and muscles, and improves cardiovascular fitness, therefore helping your paddle-power and overall surf fitness. Running also strengthens your core stability muscles, ligaments and joints, which helps your balance and rotation. Surfing a lot can result in tight neck, back and shoulders, and running can help loosen up these areas.

Running style

Get your running technique right and maximise the efficiency of every step you take. Take note of our top running tips, and you can also watch YouTube videos of the world's best runners to check out their style:

1. **Start with your head and focus on keeping it still while you run.** Continue down to your chest and hips, trying to keep your whole torso straight in line with your head. This is called running upright.
2. **Pump your arms from your chest to your hips and use them to get momentum.** Think of them as being on a train track and keep your elbows tucked in so you don't have chicken wings.
3. **Concentrate on running smoothly across the ground with minimal bounce.** You want to be flexible but strong to ensure a really good spring off the ground.

Route planning

Find a few places that you love to run. Use Google maps, Strava or the Map My Run app to check distances, and ensure that they are safe routes by driving them or running with a friend the first few times. If you're not confident of the distance or terrain, try starting at a local oval or beach where the surface is flat and the distance is easy to measure.

Stay motivated

Think big, set goals and set out to achieve them. Make sure that every time you run you are pushing yourself and moving towards your goals. Keep a motivational quote on your phone screen saver, a book about an awesome sports person by your bedside table or inspirational post-it notes on your computer. Sign up for one of the runs in your area so you are locked into an event and your goal is real. When your run gets difficult – and it will – count your steps instead of concentrating on how far you have to go. Before you know it you will be almost finished.

Listen to music

Make killer music mixes to pump you up whilst running.

Stretch

Before and after your run. Do lots of glute and hamstring stretches as those muscles get a huge workout when running.

Prevent

Listen to your body, and watch for aches and pains. If you feel like you're developing a weakness visit a physio and start a strengthening exercise programme to prevent any serious injuries. Be diligent with pre-run prep and if you are just starting out ease your body into the distance and pace.

Training drills

1. **Agility** – To improve agility whilst running you can do drills like high knees, bum kicks, knee to chest jumps and ladder running.
2. **Speed** – Intervals are a great way to improve speed – for example run for 1 minute at high intensity, then 30 seconds at an easy pace. Repeat 10 times with 5 minutes' warm up or cool down.
3. **Strength** – Stair running really helps build leg strength, or you can do weight specific gym training such as squats, lunges and calf raises to build your running muscles.

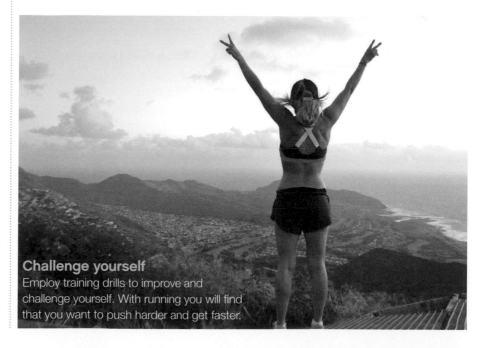

Challenge yourself
Employ training drills to improve and challenge yourself. With running you will find that you want to push harder and get faster.

5

❋

get swim fit

SWIM YOURSELF TO SURF FITNESS WITH THESE BASIC SWIMMING
PROGRAMMES FOR SURFING STRENGTH.

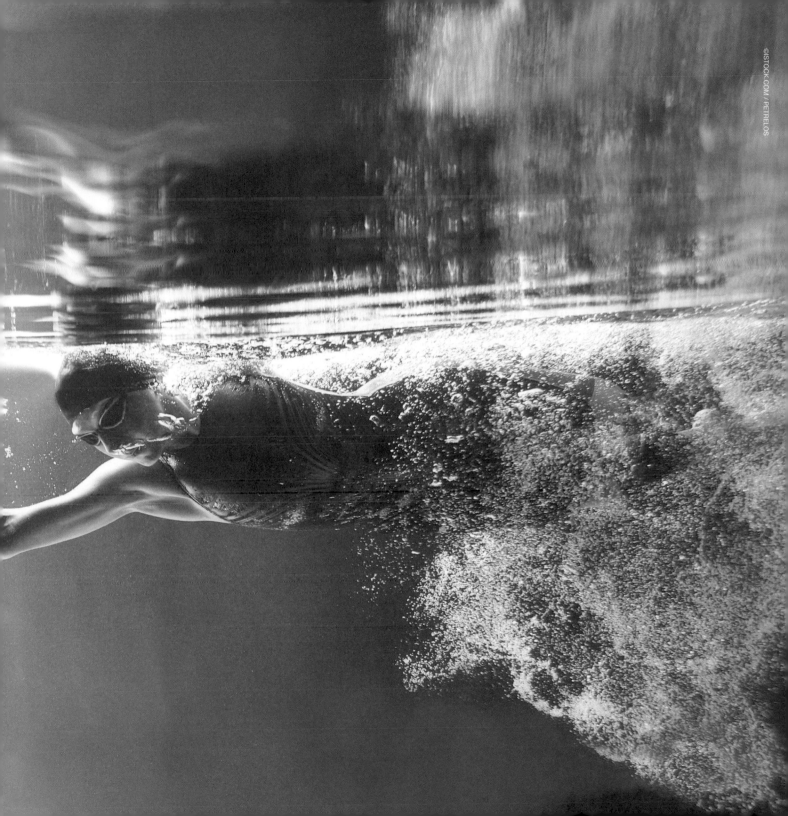

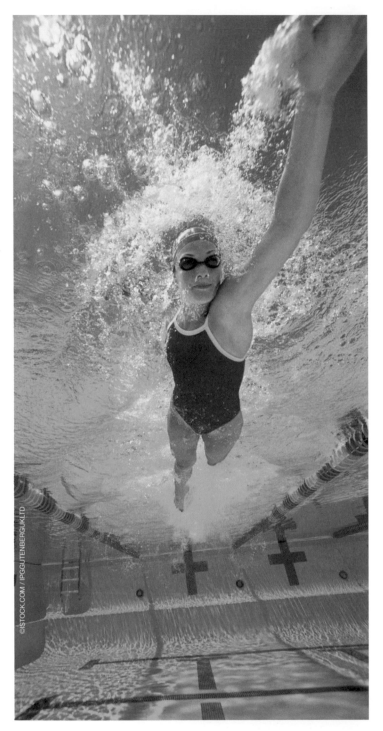

©ISTOCK.COM / IPGGUTENBERGUKLTD

SWIMMING IS ONE OF THE BEST WAYS TO IMPROVE YOUR SURF FITNESS. THE SIMPLE FACT THAT SWIMMING MOVEMENTS ARE SO SIMILAR TO PADDLING MEANS THAT A SWIM TRAINING PROGRAMME IS GUARANTEED TO BOOST YOUR SURFING FITNESS, AND SWIMMING 2-3 TIMES A WEEK CAN MAKE A MASSIVE DIFFERENCE TO YOUR PADDLE POWER. BREATH HOLDING TRAINING CAN ALSO BE USED TO PREPARE YOU FOR HOLD-DOWNS BENEATH HEAVY WAVES.

How swim training will improve your surfing:

- Catch more waves, and get into waves earlier.
- Increase aerobic capacity for paddle outs.
- Higher levels of fitness to deal with any unforeseen moments, like leash snaps or bad rips.
- Higher levels of endurance for longer surfing sessions.
- Fast paddle power to make it out past sneaker sets.

A good technique will not only improve your training session but will also reduce your risk of injury. While swimming a set distance in the pool each week will be of some benefit to your surfing, a planned weekly swimming programme will help you boost your fitness levels dramatically.

If you feel that your swimming technique is not up to much and needs improvement, contact a local swimming coach for help. To increase your fitness levels more efficiently and improve your surf fitness, you need to be able to swim front crawl.

Perceived Rate of Exertion chart:

Activity	Scale	Heart Rate
At rest	1	Non-exercise heart rate
Low level activity – sitting or walking	2	Non-exercise heart rate
Normal walk	3	50% MHR low-end aerobic
Brisk walking	4	55% MHR low-end aerobic
Medium to fast paced walking	5	60% MHR low-end aerobic
Light exertion such as a gentle jog	6	65% MHR low-end aerobic
Breathing becomes more difficult	7	75% MHR mid-end aerobic
Breathing very heavily, talk just ok	8	80% MHR high-end aerobic
Sweating, talk not possible	9	85%+ MHR anaerobic +
Max effort hard to maintain	10	90-100% MHR

Warming Up

As with all of your workouts, it's essential you follow a comprehensive warm-up procedure before your swimming session.

1: **Slow mobilisation of all limbs and joints** – this will increase blood flow to all working muscles and help warm up your body temperature.

2: **Light all over body stretch** – holding each stretch for 8-10 seconds.

3. **Light swim** – this should be done without pause and should last (depending on ability) for around 10-12 minutes. For example, try a 500m swim, with each 100m getting faster by about 10%. Or start at a very low-impact aerobic swimming level and progress to a high-end aerobic swim.

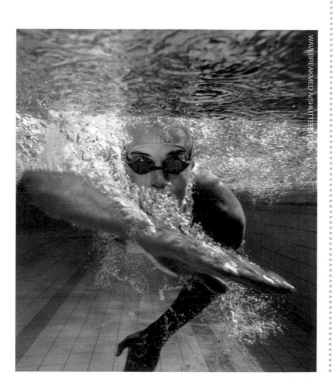

WAVEBREAKMEDIA/SHUTTERSTOCK

Target Heart Rate
To determine this number, first subtract your age from 220. This is your maximum heart rate. (MHR)

Starting Out
LOW-END AEROBIC SWIMMING

This will help you increase your swimming strength slowly but surely. If you're starting a swimming programme for the first time you should swim at a steady pace – about 60-70% of your MHR (Maximum Heart Rate) – for 30-40 minutes, 2-3 times a week for 4-6 weeks. Once you have built up your fitness levels, then it's time to introduce some basic swimming programmes.

MID-END AEROBIC TRAINING
Mid range intensity would be around 70-80% of your max HR

HIGH-END AEROBIC TRAINING
Sub maximal high level intensity would be 85%+ of your max HR

swim gear

There are several items of swim gear that can help improve your surfing and swimming strength.

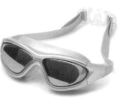
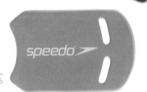
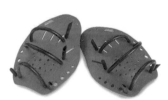
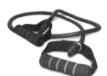
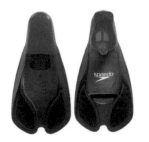
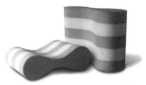

Pullbuoy

Great for improving general upper-body strength. This is placed between your legs to keeps your lower body buoyant, allowing you to pull through the water using only your upper body as you would in surfing.

Extra-large resistance bands

A great bit of kit if you can't get to the pool. These can be fixed to a solid base and used to mimic most swimming movements.

Kickboards

Kickboards allow you to target your legs, isolating them so you can practice your kick stroke, improve your balance, or work on your leg strength.

Hand paddles

Hand paddles enhance the swimmer's feel of the "catch" – the phase prior to the pull, where the hand turns from a streamlined position to grasp the water and begin the pull. If the hand catches or pulls at an incorrect angle, the increased resistance afforded by the hand paddle will exacerbate the resulting twisting moment, making the defect clearer to the swimmer.

Swim fins

Swim fins are designed to create extra resistance when kicking through the water, this builds leg strength and increases the work-rate whilst swimming.

Goggles

Swimming goggles allow you to see underwater and protect the eyes from the irritation of pool chlorine or saltwater. The goggles should be comfortable around the bridge of the nose and leave no gaps.

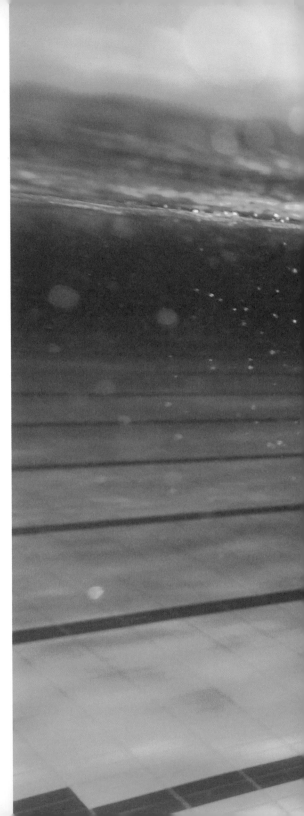

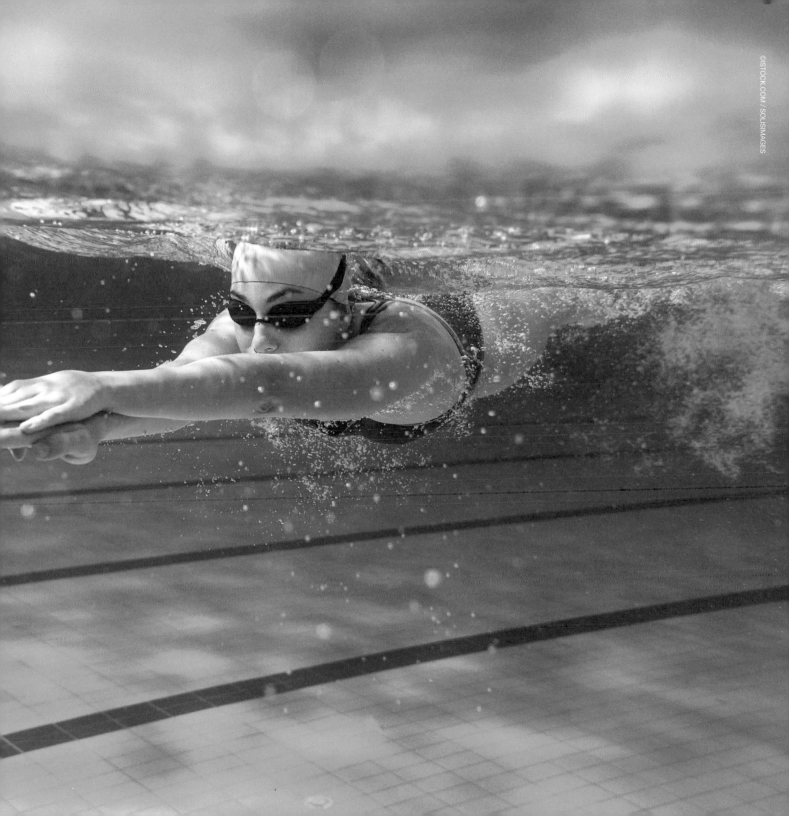

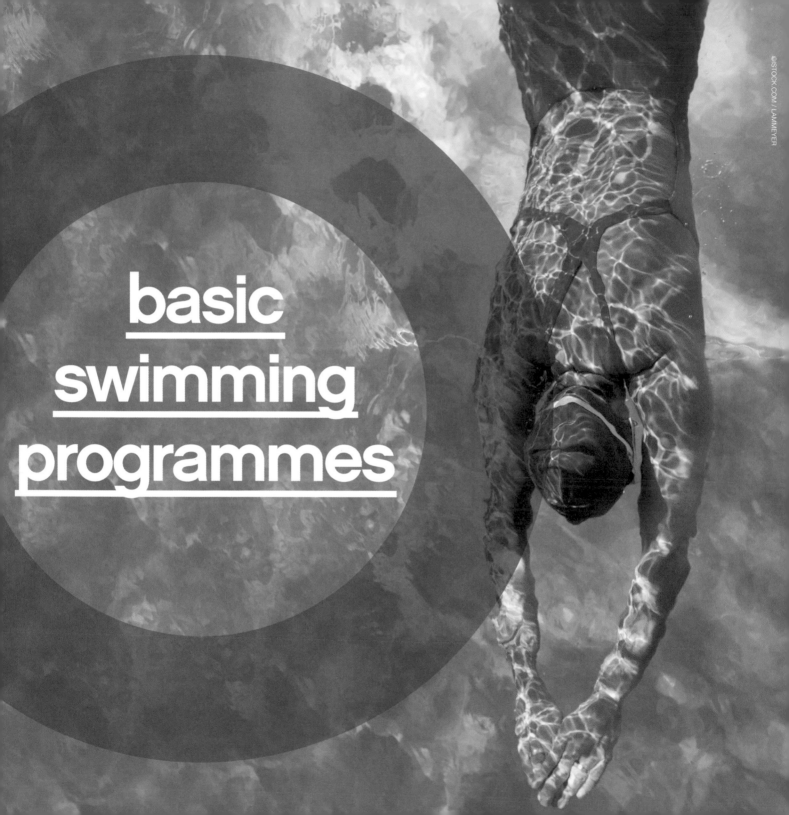

basic
swimming
programmes

The swimming distances in these programmes can be adjusted depending on your ability. If you are just starting out then start swimming short distances and slowly build up your distance as your swimming improves. Even a basic swimming programme should be progressive. Keep a record of your target times and distances, including your warm-up and cool-down sessions.

Light Aerobic

As your swimming fitness improves you will find that you are able to maintain a lower heart rate for your main session set of 12 x 50m with 10 seconds rest. Initially it may be beneficial to take a longer rest period if you are not a strong swimmer. Once you are able to do a basic distance like 400m without stopping, you may wish to add an extra 400m with the pullbuoy (with a rest interval of 60 seconds).

If your swimming fitness is very basic you will find that your heart rate will go above the low-end aerobic level during longer swims (50m+). This is normal and with regular training you will find it much easier to maintain a low heart rate.

Basic Kick Set

If you're able to complete basic swimming training on a regular weekly basis, kicking sets will be of great benefit for developing and maintaining your technique. A good kick adds balance to your stroke and aids propulsion.

Introduce this kick set into the main session of your swim training:
- Holding a float with your arms extended, swim 4 x 25m with 10 seconds rest between each.
- Repeat this 2-3 times with an additional rest after each set.
- If you're already a competent swimmer, you can increase the kicking distance according to your ability (and increase the length of your rest time).
- If you've got a poor kick this could be down to foot position and ankle flexibility; try kicking with fins on.

Anaerobic
Target: 85-95% of your MHR

Warm Up	Main Set	Cool Down
Basic mobility: 4-5 minutes Gentle stretch: 4-5 minutes (hold stretches for 8-10 seconds)	Swim 3 x 100m front crawl with 30 seconds rest after each 100m Check your HR	Swim 500m, slow and steady with each length getting slower
Swim non-stop front crawl for 400m+, with each length getting faster	2 x 150m front crawl with 45 seconds rest after each 150m Check your HR	Stretch for 8-10 minutes, covering all major muscle groups (hold each stretch for 15-20 seconds)

You may wish to add a slow, 300-500m, low-end aerobic swim using a pull float to your main session.

Basic Sprint Set

Swim training at full speed, 100% effort (95-100% of your MHR) can be of huge benefit to any surfer. Whether you're paddling to make a sneaky set or find yourself on a fat wave, sprint training can help. Sprint training in the pool should be kept to a minimum so add small amounts to your training programme for best results – sprinting daily in the pool is not advisable.

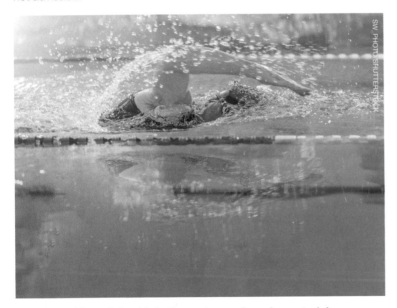

SW_PHOTO/SHUTTERSTOCK

Introduce this sprint set into the main session of your training programme:

Swim 4 x 25m front crawl, flat out with 60 seconds rest between each 25m.	Swim 4 x 25m front crawl, sprinting half of each length, with 30 seconds rest between each 25m.	Swim 4 x 25m front crawl, getting progressively faster at the end of each length.

After 2-3 weeks you may wish to progress your sprint set by adding an extra 25-50m each week.

Sprint Tips:
- Ensure you do a decent warm up
- Give yourself a week's break from sprinting every 4 weeks, for recovery.
- Do a good cool-down swim after sprint sets to aid recovery.

Swim Fitness Tests

To monitor your pool training and for additional surfing fitness, record the results from your training sessions in a weekly diary. You may also wish to test your swimming fitness levels with one of the basic swim-fit tests below:

As with any intense exercise, a constructive warm up with mobility stretches will aid performance and a cool down will aid recovery.

TEST 1: The TT (Time Trial)

This is basically a distance swim over a set time.
E.g. Swim as far as you can in 20 minutes then record the distance.

TEST 2: Basic HR (Heart Rate) Test

For the most accurate reading use a heart rate monitor.
- After warming up, swim a short set distance (e.g. 200m) as fast as you can at 100% effort.
- As soon as you finish take your HR.
- Continue to record your HR at set timed periods, to track the progress of the improvements in your recovery rate.
- Always use the same distance and cool down period for each test.
  For example:
  - Immediately after exercise, record HR
  - 30 seconds after exercise, record HR
  - 60 seconds after exercise, record HR

Keep a record of all – and of your resting HR – and repeat every four weeks.

As you get fitter your HR readings should fall and you should recover more quickly.

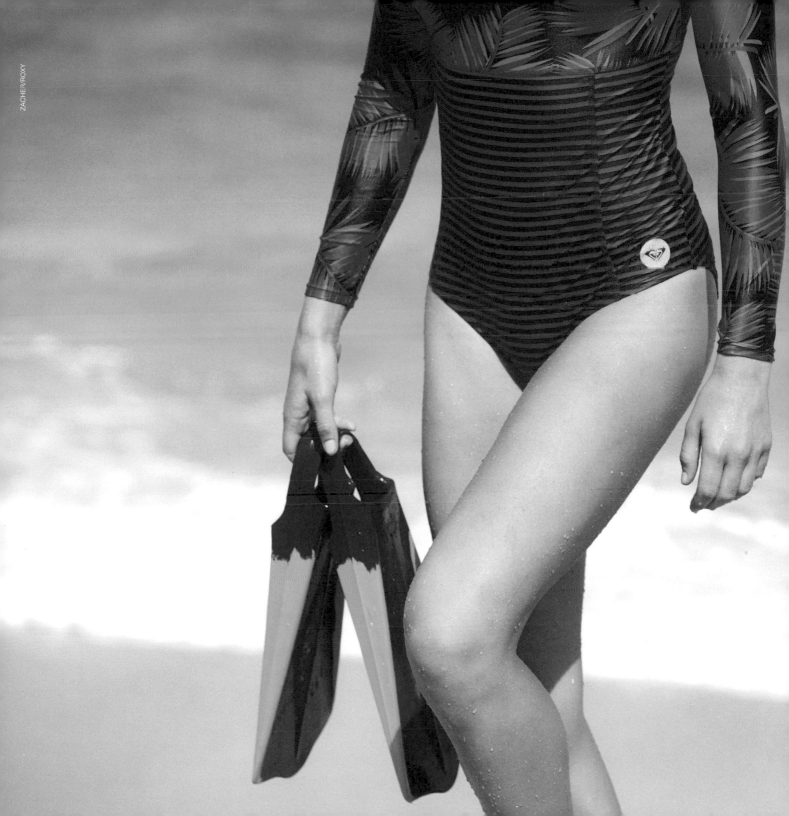

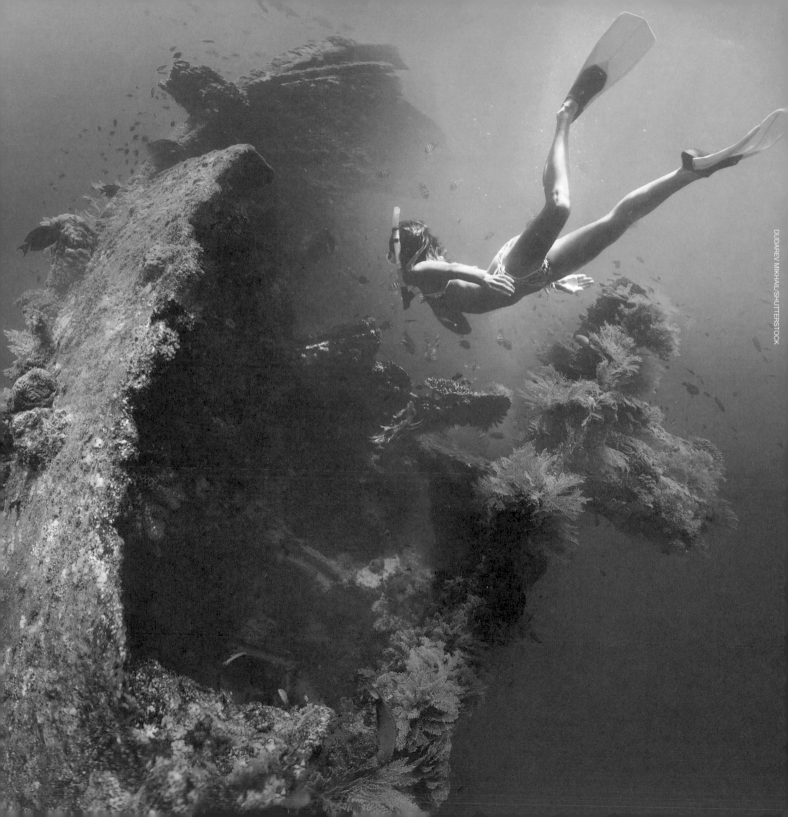

Hypoxic Swim Training (Breath Holding)

As surfers we've all experienced that hold down after getting nailed by a wave – and the feeling that you're not coming up and fast running out of air while you're being rolled around underwater like a rag doll. There is no perfect way to deal with a major hold-down or wipeout, but if you panic and increase the speed of movement, you will use up what oxygen you have left in your body even faster – causing you to panic even more.

What we really need to do during a hold-down is relax: your heart rate is slower when you are relaxed, thus your demand for oxygen decreases. However, putting this technique into practice can be easier said than done. A more practical solution is to increase your lung capacity, which will enable you to take on increased levels of oxygen and give you valuable extra seconds underwater. Breath holding in a pool can help you prepare, and is known as hypoxic (low oxygen) swimming training.

Hypoxic training was developed some years ago and can significantly help swimmers to maintain a smooth stroke when the pressure is on over a set racing distance. Or in your case, help make the inevitable hold down less daunting.

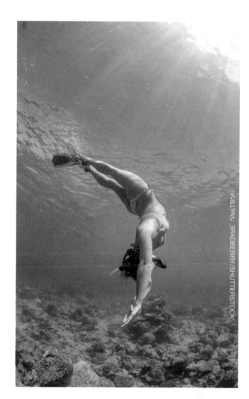

5-week Hypoxic Training Programme – to prepare you for that inevitable hold-down.

Week	Week 1	Week 2	Week 3	Week 4	Week 5
SwimSet Breakdown	2 sets of 12 x 25m front crawl 10 seconds rest after each 25m length 60 seconds rest after 12 lengths	2 sets of 12 x 25m front crawl 10 seconds rest after each 25m length 60 seconds rest after 12 lengths	2 sets of 12 x 25m front crawl 10 seconds rest after each 25m length 60 seconds rest after 12 lengths	2 sets of 12 x 25m front crawl 10 seconds rest after each 25m length 60 seconds rest after 12 lengths	2 sets of 12 x 25m front crawl 10 seconds rest after each 25m length 60 seconds rest after 12 lengths
Breathing Rate	Every 4 strokes	Every 5 strokes	Every 6 strokes	Every 7 strokes	Every 8 strokes

A good way to test your progress during a hypoxic training programme is to swim as far as you can underwater every few weeks and record the distance. **If you are new to swimming then extra care should be taken with any breath holding exercises. You need to begin each session with a stretch and warm-up swim.**

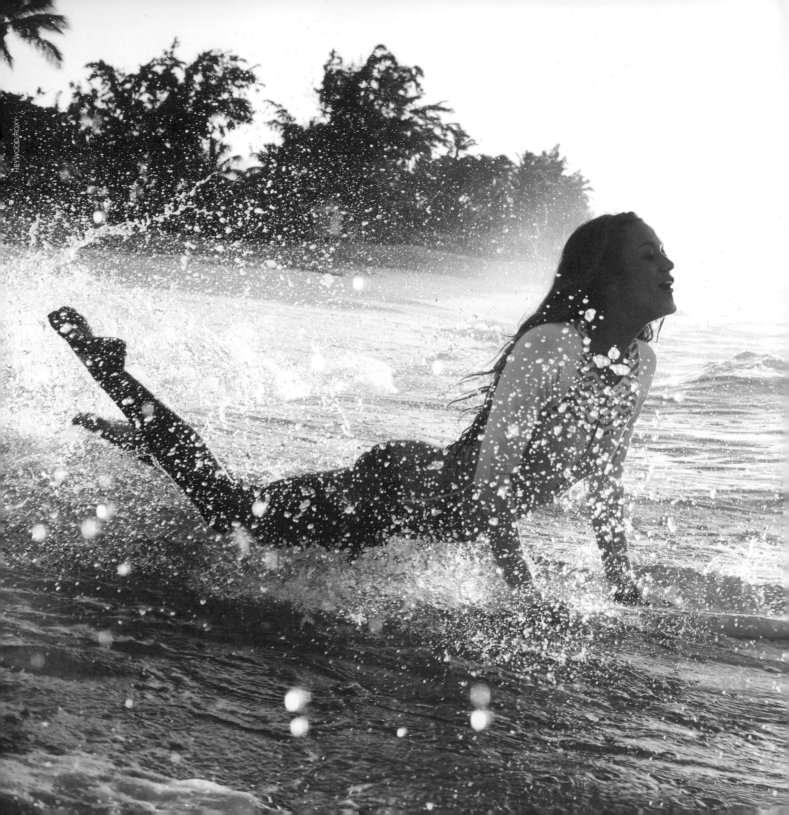

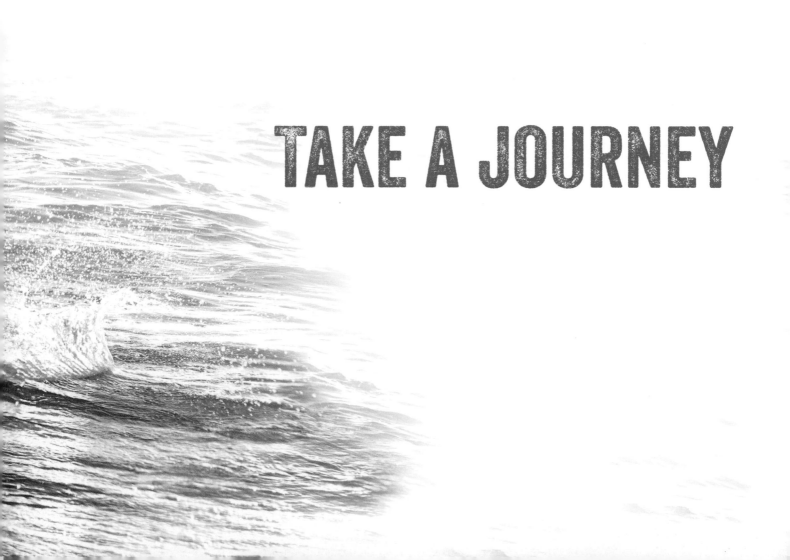

TAKE A JOURNEY

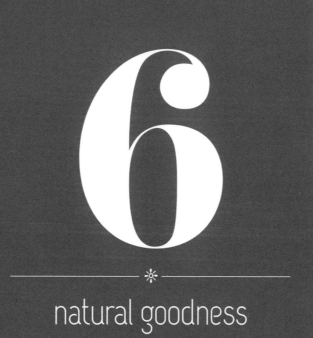

6

natural goodness

YOU NEED TO BE IN GOOD HEALTH TO REALLY PUSH YOUR SURFING AND A BIG PART OF THAT IS BEING CAREFUL ABOUT WHAT YOU PUT INTO YOUR BODY. WHOLESOME, NATURAL FOODS WILL NOURISH YOU ON EVERY LEVEL.

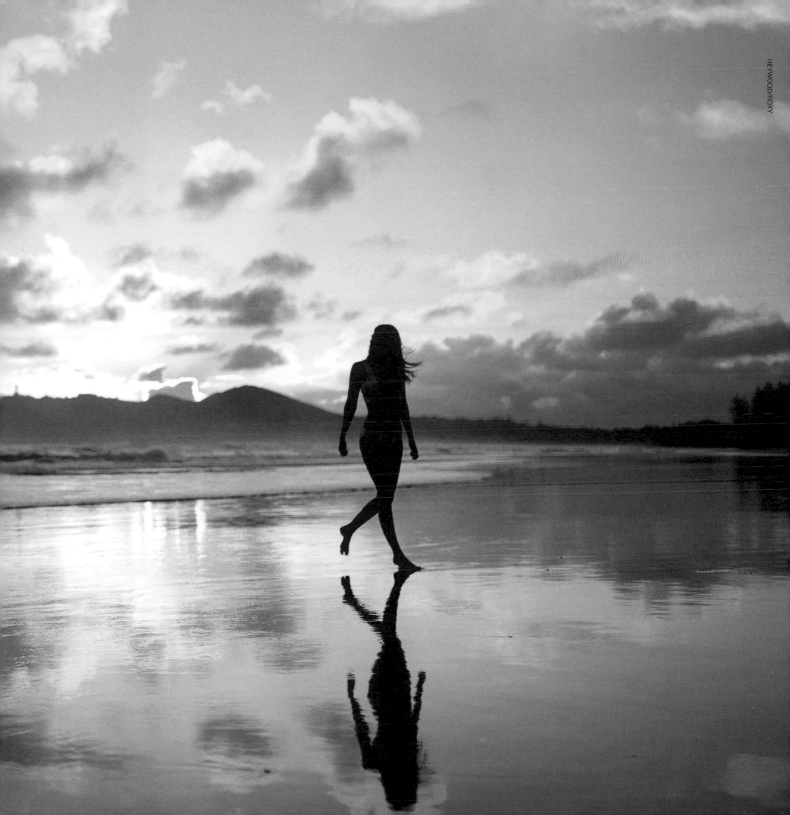

eat well

Tired of diets and failed healthy eating resolutions, but want to do something to improve your lifestyle and eating habits? It's time to turn good intentions into reality. These tips and recipe suggestions from Samantha Bass, a qualified naturopath and specialist in holistic nutrition, use all natural, wholesome, functional foods. Sam says: "Being a surfer myself I know that the nutritional demands are high, and I know how much better I feel out in the surf after eating the right foods." Give Sam's recipes a go and energise your body ready for your surf sessions.

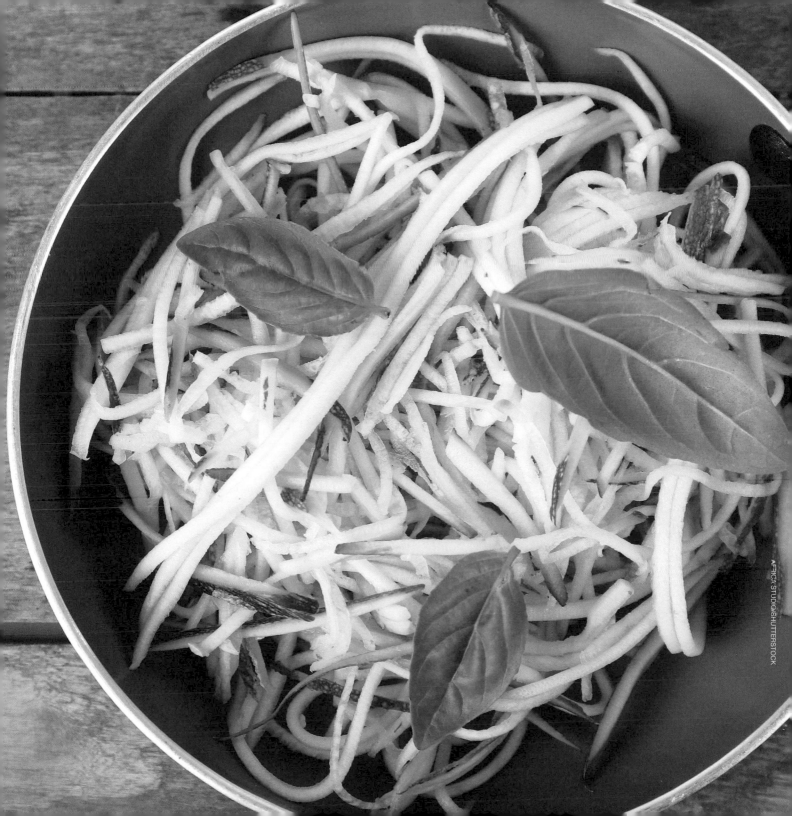

breakfast

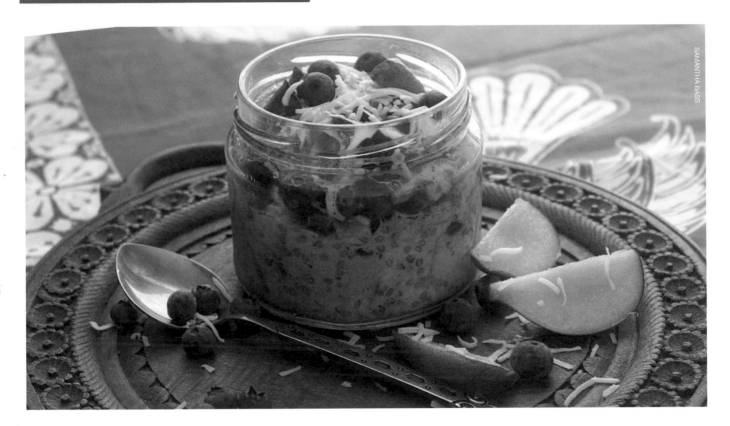

SAMANTHA BASS

Chia Oat Pudding

Ingredients *(Serves 2)*
- 1 cup rolled oats
- 2 tbsp chia seeds
- 1 grated apple
- 2 tbsp goji berries
- 2 cups almond milk, to cover (or milk of choice)
- Pinch of cinnamon
- Honey, fresh fruit and desiccated coconut to serve

Method
- Prepare the night before.
- In a container mix the chia seeds, oats, apple, goji berries and cinnamon.
- Generously pour the milk over the mixture until it is completely covered and stir through (the ingredients will absorb the milk so make sure there is a little extra).
- Put it in the fridge overnight.
- To serve, top with fresh fruit, desiccated coconut and honey. Add some extra milk if desired.

What is it good for?
Preparing it the night before makes this Chia Oat Pudding a quick, easy breakfast before hitting the waves early. It's thought that chia seeds were so highly valued by the Aztecs as a food that they were also used as currency. The combination of oats and chia seeds provides a balance of protein, complex carbs, fibre and omega 3 fats, helping to keep you fuller for longer and provide sustained energy.

Green Eggs with Sourdough Toast

Ingredients *(Serves 2)*

- 4 eggs (free-range or organic are best)
- 2 cups baby kale leaves, chopped
- 2 tbsp green shallots, chopped
- 2 tbsp parsley, chopped
- 2 tbsp feta cheese, crumbled
- Dash of milk
- Olive oil for cooking
- Celtic sea salt and fresh cracked pepper, to taste
- Sourdough toast for serving

Method

- Whisk the eggs and milk in a bowl.
- Heat the olive oil in a skillet on medium heat. Add the kale leaves, stirring whilst they cook. Once the kale leaves have wilted add the eggs, stirring to scramble.
- Once the eggs are almost cooked add the shallots and feta, stirring through for another minute.
- To serve, sprinkle parsley over the top and add salt and pepper to taste.
- Serve with toast if desired.

What is it good for?

Eggs are a powerhouse of nutrients including protein, vitamins A, D, E and B, minerals, iodine, zinc and calcium. Many of these nutrients are only found in the yolk, so skip the 'egg white only' fad because these nutrients are extremely important. Interestingly, eggs may help prevent macula degeneration (a common eye complaint of older surfers) due to their high levels of carotenoids, lutein and zeaxanthin. Eating high protein foods like eggs in the morning can also help to reduce sugar cravings later in the day.

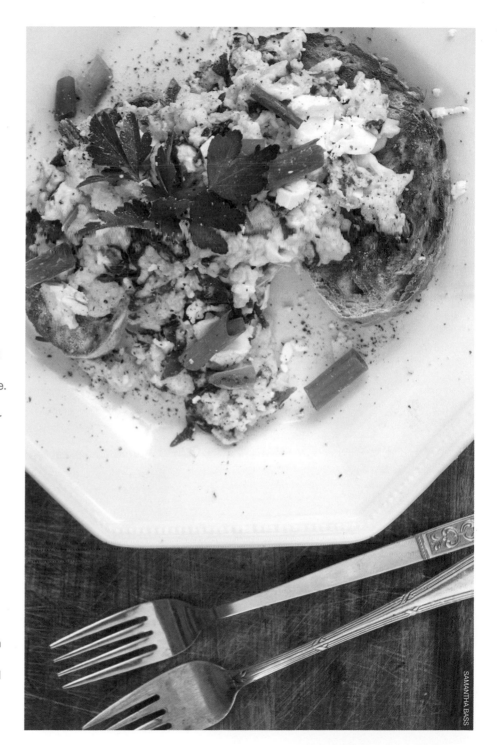

SAMANTHA BASS

lunch

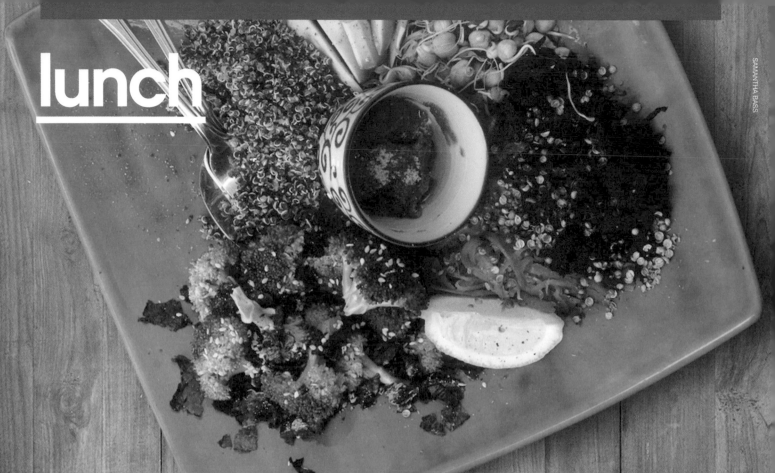

Zen Macrobiotic Plate

Ingredients *(Serves 2)*
- ½ cup quinoa
- 1/3 cup mixed sprouts
- 1 seaweed sheet, sliced into thin, short strips
- 1 tbsp sesame seeds
- ½ cup broccoli, lightly steamed
- ½ avocado
- ½ carrot, grated
- ½ beetroot, grated
- 1 tsp crushed coriander seed

Tahini dressing
- 2 tbsp tahini
- Juice of ¼ lemon
- Cracked black pepper

Method

Quinoa
- Rinse the quinoa to remove the bitter coating.
- Bring to the boil ½ cup quinoa with 1 cup water in an uncovered pot.
- Cover, turn the heat to low and allow it to simmer for about 15 minutes until the water has been absorbed (check intermittently to ensure it doesn't dry out).
- Remove from the heat once all of the water is absorbed and the quinoa is soft and chewy.

Tahini dressing
- Mix the tahini and lemon in a small bowl, adding pepper to taste. For a thinner consistency add a little water.

To serve
- Use the sesame seeds and seaweed to sprinkle over the steamed broccoli.
- The broccoli and quinoa can be prepared the night before, making it easy to pop it in a container to take to work or on a day trip.

What is it good for?
The term macrobiotic comes from Greek roots and can be translated to mean 'long life'. The macrobiotic philosophy is one of a simple diet to support health and reduce disease. The incorporation of vegetarian meals into your daily diet can help to boost fibre and antioxidant levels, assisting the body's detoxification processes.

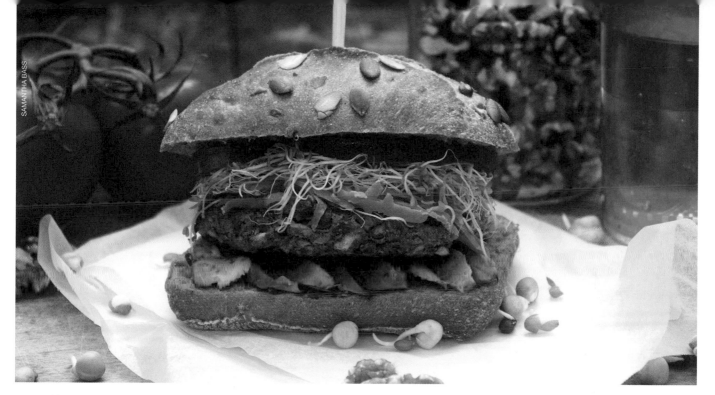

Walnut Burger

Ingredients *(Makes 6 patties)*
Walnut patties
- ¾ cup walnuts, toasted
- 1 tin lentils, drained
- ½ cup fresh breadcrumbs
- 1 egg
- ½ onion, finely chopped
- 2 cloves garlic, crushed
- 1 tbsp fresh oregano, chopped
- 1 tbsp fresh parsley, chopped
- Celtic sea salt and cracked pepper to taste
- Olive oil for cooking

To serve
- Buns
- 1 avocado
- ½ cup alfalfa sprouts
- 1 carrot, grated
- 1 tomato, sliced
- Peanut sauce

Method
- Lightly toast the walnuts in a hot, dry skillet until they have darkened but aren't burnt.
- Crush the walnuts.
- In a food processor, blend the lentils, breadcrumbs, onion, garlic and herbs.
- Transfer to a bowl and stir through with the egg and walnuts. Season the mix with salt and pepper.
- Spoon out small portions of the mixture to shape into palm-size patties.
- Warm the oil in a medium-hot skillet and cook the patties for 5 minutes or until firm and the undersides have turned medium brown. Then flip and cook the other side for another 5 minutes. Cut one in half to make sure it is cooked through.
- Serve hot on a bun with salads.
- The patties can be frozen and reheated at work for a yummy, healthy lunch.

What is it good for?
Walnuts not only make the veggie patties delicious, they also increase the nutritional value of the dish by supplying magnesium and zinc – two of the most common deficiencies of people living in developed countries. We need both of these essential minerals for adequate energy levels, muscle function and sleep.

dinner

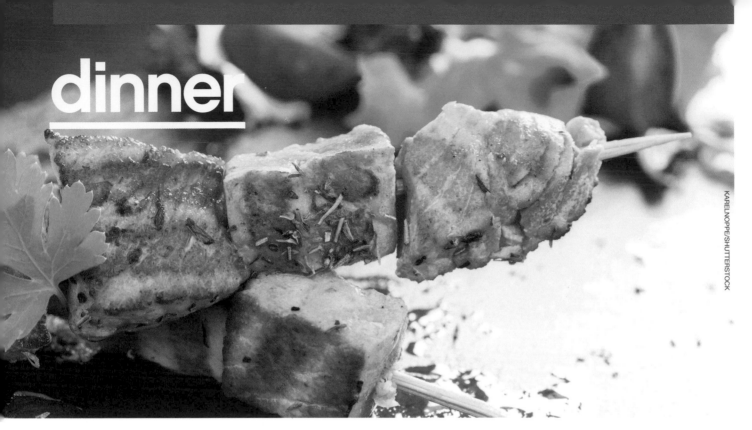

Tuna Skewers with Courgette Couscous

Ingredients *(Serves 2)*

- 2 tuna steaks (sustainably sourced*), chopped into 2cm squares
- 2 garlic cloves, chopped
- ½ large fresh red chilli, chopped
- ½ lemon, zested
- 1 cup couscous
- 1 fennel bulb, thinly sliced
- 1 punnet cherry tomatoes, halved
- 2 courgettes, sliced lengthways
- ½ avocado, chopped
- ¼ cup olive oil
- Celtic sea salt and cracked pepper to taste
- 6 skewers

Method

- Mix the olive oil, garlic, chilli and lemon zest in a bowl.
- Soak the chopped tuna in the marinade for 10-30 minutes.
- Warm olive oil on a grill plate and brown the courgette strips on each side – this should only take a few minutes.
- Remove from the heat and put aside.
- Cook the couscous according to instructions on the packet.
- Mix the couscous, fennel, tomatoes, avocado and courgette into a salad.
- Slide the tuna chunks onto skewers (leaving space in between each chunk so they cook properly.)
- Cook the tuna skewers on the hot grill plate for about 4 minutes on each side, or until nicely browned.

What is it good for?

Tuna is high in omega 3 fatty acids, which support health, concentration, metabolism, skin texture and circulation. The addition of fennel to the salad assists with digestion, as fennel is traditionally used to reduce bloating and stomach cramps.

* Choose line and pole caught tuna, as this more sustainable method of fishing is less likely to cause harm to other marine species. Also bear in mind that bigeye and yellowfin tuna are species under threat, so it's best to choose other types of tuna.

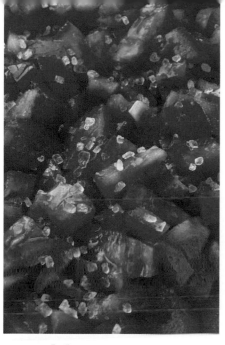

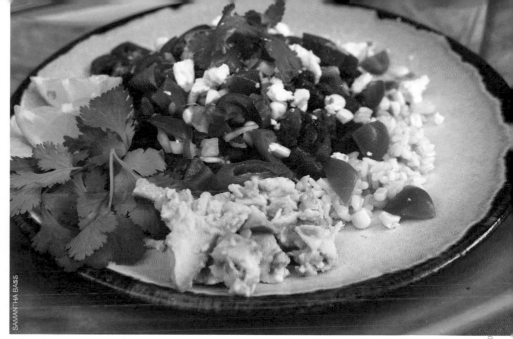

SAMANTHA BASS

Healthy Mexican Bowl

Ingredients *(Serves 2)*
- 1 cup brown rice
- 1 can kidney beans
- ½ can chopped tomatoes
- 1 clove garlic, crushed
- 1 tsp cumin seeds
- 1 tsp paprika
- 1 tbsp fresh oregano, chopped
- ½ large fresh chilli, chopped
- 1 tbsp olive oil for cooking

Salsa
- 1 punnet cherry tomatoes, finely chopped
- ¼ red onion, finely chopped
- ½ green capsicum, finely chopped
- 1 fresh corn on the cob, kernels sliced off
- Juice of ½ lemon

To serve
- Fresh coriander, chopped
- 1 avocado, mashed
- Jalapeno

Method
- Bring to the rice to boil with 2 cups water in an uncovered pot.
- Cover, turn the heat to low and allow it to simmer for about 15 minutes or until all of the water has been absorbed and the rice is soft and chewy (check it intermittently to ensure it doesn't dry out).
- For the mexi beans, warm the oil in a hot skillet, add the garlic, cumin seeds, paprika, oregano and chilli, stir and cook until aromatic.
- Add the kidney beans, stirring. Then add the tomatoes and stir. Cook for a few minutes until all ingredients are mixed.
- Mix the salsa ingredients together in a bowl, squeezing the lemon juice on at the end and stirring through.
- To serve, arrange the rice, mexi beans and salsa in a bowl and top with avocado, coriander and jalapenos.

Why is it good?
This veggie meal follows protein-combining principals, with brown rice and kidney beans ensuring a complete range of amino acids are in the meal. While white rice is generally more popular than brown rice, wholegrain brown rice is lower in GI, contains more protein and is higher in B vitamins. Brown rice also tends to keep you fuller for longer, making it a good option for active people.

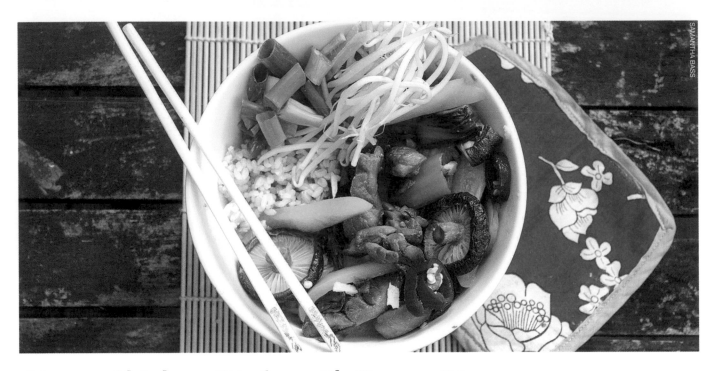

Ginger Chicken Stir-fry with Brown Rice

Ingredients *(Serves 2)*
- 300g chicken thigh fillets, sliced (free range, organic if possible)
- 1 bunch bok choy, chopped
- 1 pepper, chopped
- 4 shitake mushrooms, fresh or re-hydrated and sliced
- 1 large chilli, chopped
- 2 garlic cloves, crushed
- 1 tbsp fresh ginger, sliced
- 2 green shallots, chopped
- ¼ cup tamari sauce
- 1/3 cup water
- 2 tbsp sesame seeds
- 1 cup brown rice
- Olive oil
- 1 cup bean shoots

Method
- Bring the rice and 2 cups water to the boil in an uncovered pot. Cover, turn the heat to low and simmer for about 15 minutes until the rice has absorbed the water and the rice is soft and chewy (check intermittently to ensure it doesn't dry out). Remove from the heat.
- Make the marinade by mixing the tamari sauce, water, half of the garlic, half of the chilli and half of the ginger in a bowl. Pour over chicken and leave for 5-10 minutes.
- Warm the oil in a hot wok and add the chicken, allowing it to seal for a couple of minutes. Put the chicken aside.
- Add the rest of the chilli, ginger and garlic to the wok and cook until aromatic (less than a minute), then add the bok choy, pepper and shitake mushrooms, and stir fry for a minute or so.
- Add the chicken and an extra dash of tamari and water. Continue stir-frying for a couple of minutes to allow the chicken to cook through and the veggies to soften but still have some crunch.
- Top with sesame seeds, spring onions and bean shoots.

What is it good for?
This nutritious meal is the perfect dinner after a day of surfing. Chicken is a good source of glutamine, an amino acid that is important for muscle repair and growth. The ginger and chilli both help to reduce inflammation, which is the one of the main causes of post exercise muscle soreness. The meal also possesses a broad range of support for the immune system, as the shitake mushrooms increase immune cell activity, pepper provides vitamin C and garlic kills off harmful bacteria.

Wasabi Salmon with Wedges

Ingredients *(Serves 2)*

- 2 fresh salmon steaks (sustainably fished)
- 5 potatoes, chopped into wedges
- 1 bunch of broccolini (hybrid of broccoli and chard), stalk removed
- ½ bunch kale, stems removed, roughly chopped
- 1 handful of green beans
- ½ tsp wasabi paste
- 3cm piece ginger, finely chopped
- 1 garlic clove, crushed
- ¼ tsp lemon zest

Method

- Preheat the oven to 180C.
- Chop the potato into chunky wedges, sprinkle with olive oil and toss to coat evenly. Bake in the oven for 45 minutes or until golden and crispy on the outside.
- Grind the ginger, garlic and lemon zest with pestle and mortar. Thinly spread the paste along the fleshy underside of the salmon. Place in an oven pan lined with baking paper, skin side down and bake for 30 minutes or until lightly browned and cooked through.
- Steam the greens for 15 minutes or until they reach desired softness.
- Serve wasabi paste on the side and spread desired amount onto salmon.

What is it good for?

The healthy version of fish and chips! Get good quality protein and omega 3s from the salmon and replenish carbohydrate levels with oven-baked potato wedges. Wasabi is one of Asia's superfoods and is great for clearing the sinuses, as well as assisting with liver detoxification along with the kale, broccolini, garlic and lemon. The kale and broccolini are also sources of iron and calcium. Squeezing fresh lemon juice over the greens will make the iron be more easily absorbed.

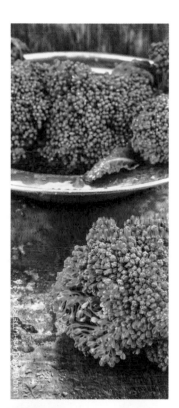

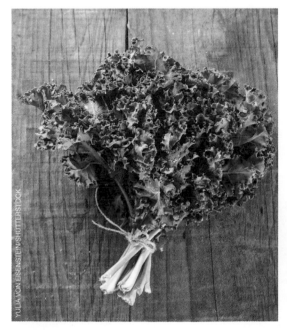

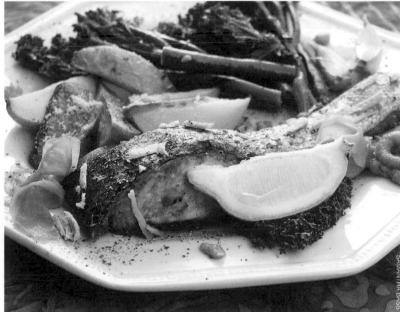

post-surf snack

These flax crackers help to restore protein levels after surfing. Topping them with banana also helps replenish carbohydrates and the seeds contain high levels of vitamins, minerals, omega 3 and omega 6. It's best to use is Celtic sea salt, as it contains a wide range of trace minerals compared to regular table salt that is often highly processed and can result in the loss of different minerals.

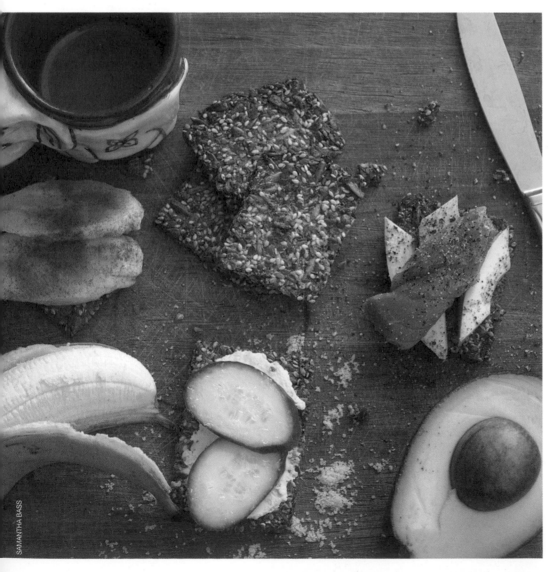

SAMANTHA BASS

Seedy Flax Crackers

Ingredients
- ½ cup flaxseeds
- ½ cup sunflower seeds
- ½ cup sesame seeds
- ¾ cup almond meal
- 250ml water
- ¼ tsp Celtic sea salt

Method
- Preheat oven to 160C.
- Mix all of the ingredients in a bowl. Let it sit for a few minutes to absorb all of the water.
- Line a baking tray with baking paper and thinly spread the mixture into the tray using the back of a spoon, making it about 5mm thick. Bake for 30 minutes.
- Take them out of the oven, cut into desirable sizes, flip the crackers over and bake for another 25 minutes.
- Allow the crackers to cool (they can be stored in the fridge for a couple of weeks).

Serve with:
- Banana and cinnamon
- Ricotta cheese and cucumber
- Avocado and smoked salmon

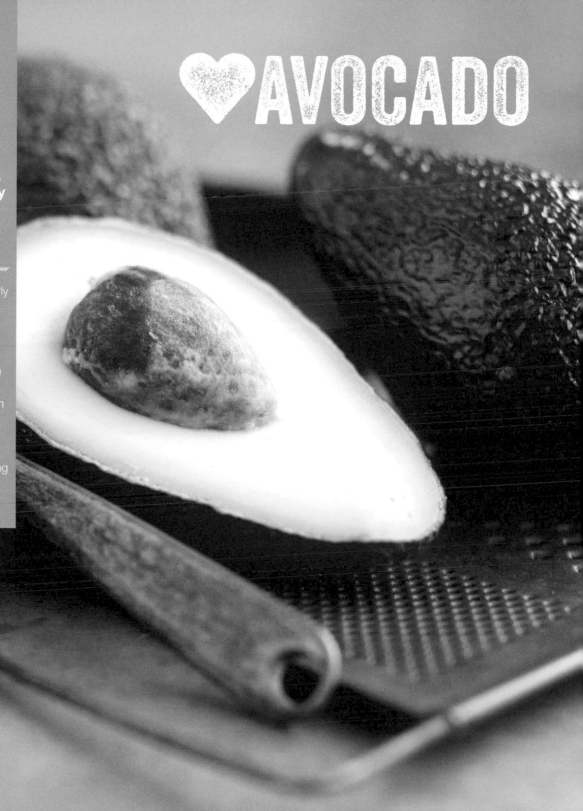

♥AVOCADO

The avocado is right up there at the top when it comes to heart healthy foods. Avocados have been shown to lower bad cholesterol (LDL) while raising your good cholesterol (HDL) levels, plus they help your body absorb heart-healthy vitamins such as beta-carotene and lycopene.

Avocado eaters have significantly higher intakes of certain nutrients, including 48% more vitamin K, 36% more fibre, 23% more vitamin E, 16% more potassium and 13% more magnesium. Avocados can lower your BMI and they contain healthy (monounsaturated and polyunsaturated) fats. By eating these super fruits, you have up to 50% lower odds of developing metabolic syndrome, a group of risk factors for heart disease, diabetes, and stroke.

super smoothies

Whizz together these nutritious ingredients to kick-start your energy levels and boost your immune system

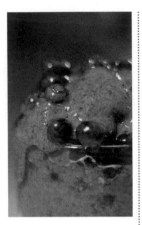

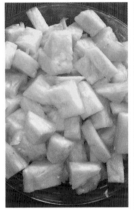

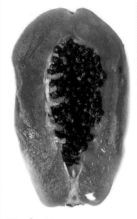

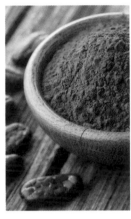

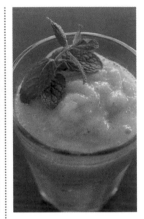

Red Glow Girl

- 1 cup green tea
- 1 cup mixed frozen berries
- 1 tbsp goji berries
- 1 tbsp flaxseeds
- Juice of ½ orange

BENEFITS:
- Boosts antioxidant levels
- Source of Vitamin C and bioflavonoids
- Anti-inflammatory properties

Pineapple Mint Lassi

- 1½ cups chopped pineapple
- ½ cup natural probiotic yoghurt (runny ones work best)
- ¼ cup water
- 10 fresh mint leaves
- 1/3 cup coconut milk

BENEFITS:
- Reduces inflammation and supports the healing of injuries
- Supports healthy digestion with good bacteria
- Source of Calcium

Hydrating Green Blast

- 1½ cups coconut water
- 1 cup baby spinach
- 1 cup papaya, chopped
- 2 kiwi fruits, peeled
- 1/3 cup cashews
- 1 cucumber, peeled
- Juice of ½ lime
- Pinch of Celtic sea salt

BENEFITS:
- Re-hydrating and supplies electrolytes
- Rich in a range of vitamins and minerals
- Provides antioxidants

Restorative Cacao Thick-Shake

- 1 tbsp protein powder
- 1 tbsp cacao powder
- ½ tsp vanilla essence
- 1 banana, chopped
- 1 cup almond milk
- ½ tbsp Ashwagandha powder (optional)
- 2 tbsp oats
- Pinch of nutmeg, freshly grated

BENEFITS:
- Restores protein and carbohydrate levels after a workout
- Supports healthy brain and nervous system function
- Keeps energy levels up

Mango Spice

- 1 cup mango
- 1 cup milk of choice
- ½ tbsp tahini
- ½ tbsp chia seeds
- ½ tsp turmeric
- 1 tsp fresh ginger, grated
- 1 tsp vanilla essence

BENEFITS:
- Anti-inflammatory components help reduce pain and inflammation
- Rich in essential fatty acids
- Good source of fibre

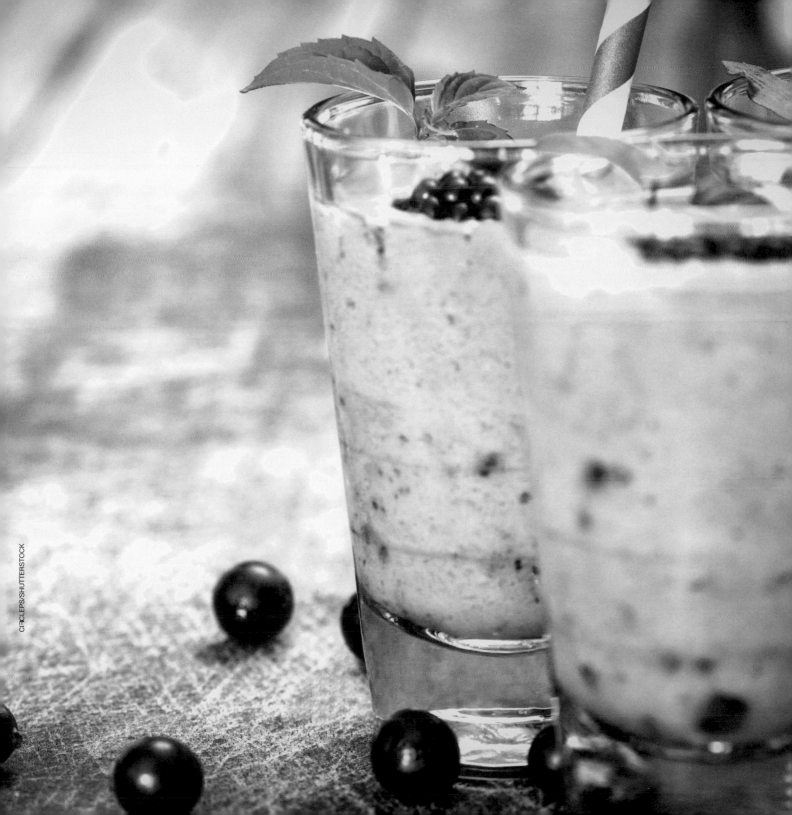

green smoothies

Green smoothies are the best way to kick-start your day on a healthy note. Naturally-occurring in vitamins, minerals and antioxidants, these easy and quick smoothies give you plenty of energy to get you through an energetic surf session (no need for coffee.) and contain daily servings of fruits and vegetables.

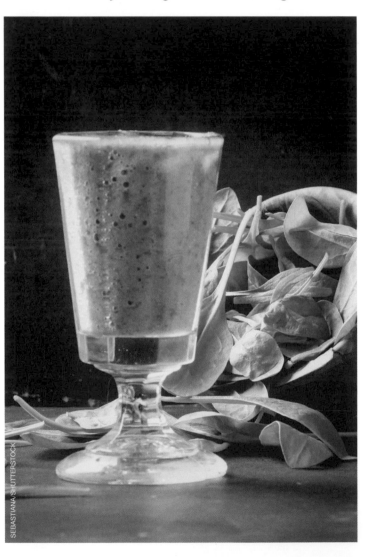

SEBASTIANA /SHUTTERSTOCK

The Green Berry
- 4 large pieces of kale
- 1 banana
- Almond milk
- 2 cups of your favourite berries

BOOST IT UP:
Chia seeds – contain good balance of high quality proteins and essential amino acids for your body and brain.

The Green Supreme
- 2 cups of fresh spinach
- Coconut water
- 1 banana
- 1 apple
- Half a pineapple

BOOST IT UP:
Acai powder – the extract instantly increases overall levels of energy and stamina.

The Green Vitamix
- Wheatgrass powder
- Lime juice
- 1 kiwi
- 1 apple
- 15 grapes

BOOST IT UP:
Flax seeds – not only rich in essential healthy omega3, these also offer plenty of minerals and vitamins.

Meal Plan

Feel great and put some of our recipes to the test with this 3-day meal plan

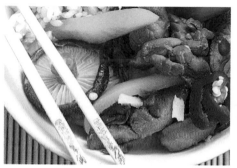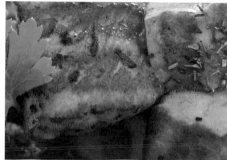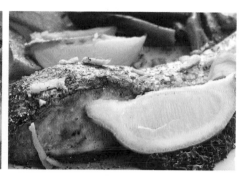

Day 1

Rising:	Juice of ½ lemon in 250ml glass of water
Breakfast:	Chia oat pudding, green tea
Morning Surf/ workout Post-surf snack:	Mango spice smoothie, extra water to rehydrate
Lunch:	Zen macro bowl, glass of water
Afternoon tea:	Seedy flax crackers with avocado, glass of coconut water
Dinner:	Ginger chicken stir-fry with brown rice, glass of water
Optional desert:	Couple of squares of dark chocolate, passionflower tea

Day 2

Rising:	Juice of ½ lemon in 250ml glass of water
Breakfast:	Green eggs with sour dough toast, green tea
Morning Surf/ workout Post-surf snack:	Glow girl smoothie
Lunch:	Walnut burger, glass of water
Afternoon tea:	2 Iron woman herbal energy balls, rosehip tea
Dinner:	Tuna skewers with couscous salad, glass of water
Optional desert:	Small tub of natural yoghurt, passionflower tea

Day 3

Rising:	Juice of ½ lemon in 250ml glass of water
Breakfast:	Restorative cacao thick-shake
Morning Surf/ workout Post-surf snack:	Seedy flax crackers with ricotta and cucumber, bottle of water to rehydrate
Lunch:	Zen macro bowl, glass of water
Afternoon tea:	Piece of fruit, green tea
Dinner:	Wasabi baked salmon with wedges, glass of water
Optional desert:	Seedy cracker with banana, honey and cinnamon, passionflower tea

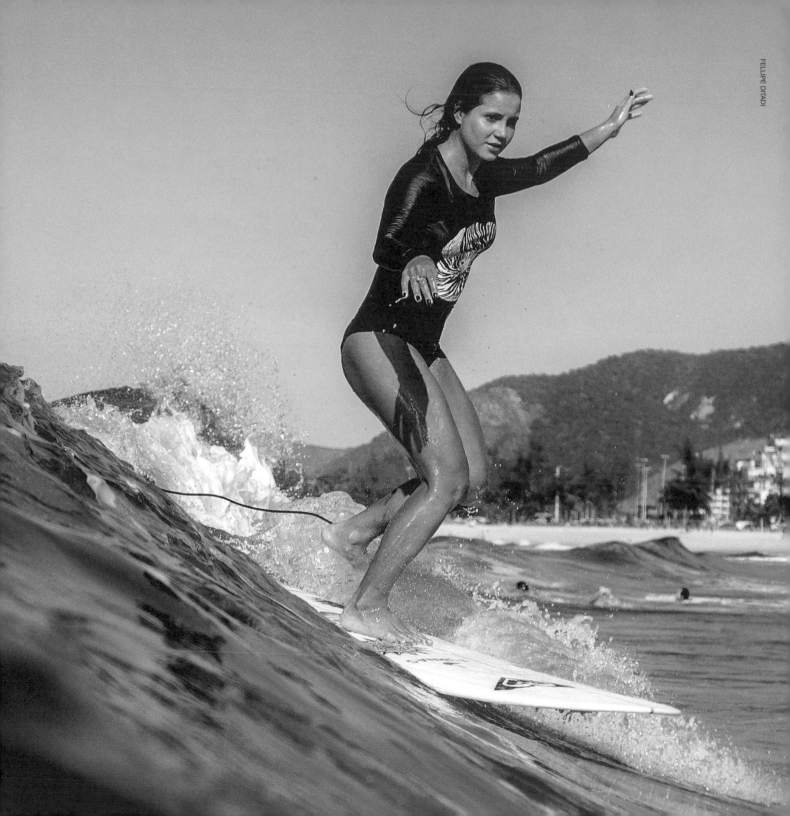

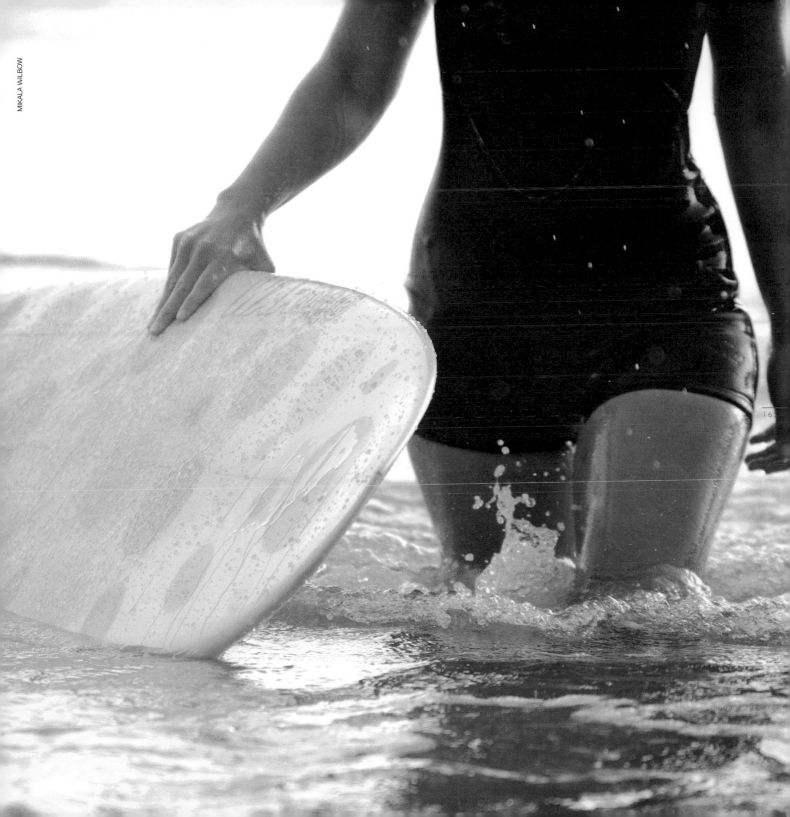

healthy
herbs
for Active Women

For centuries herbs have been used to support health and vitality. While a nutritional diet, exercise and rest are essential for maintaining health and energy when you lead a busy, active lifestyle, adding herbs into you daily life can help you feel more balanced and able to cope with higher levels of physical and mental demands. Densely packed with vitamins and minerals, herbs contain vital nutrients and 'phytochemicals' – active plant substances that have positive effects on the body, mind and emotions.

Surfers' Herbal Remedy Kit

Ashwagandha root
What for? Vitality
In Ayurveda, Ashwagandha is thought to be a rejuvenator for physical and mental health. Supporting mood, energy, concentration and the immune system, it's useful when your body is under increased demand, such as during intense training or workloads. It also assists adaptation to stress and supports recovery from anaemia – a common complaint of female athletes.
How do I take it?
An easy way to integrate it into your diet is to add a tablespoon of Ashwagandha powder to energy balls and smoothies.

Turmeric root
What for? Pain and inflammation
Antioxidant, anti-inflammatory, pain relieving, turmeric helps joint pain, injuries and arthritis. It also assists detoxification, digestive inflammation, and cancer prevention.
How do I take it?
Add a teaspoon of turmeric powder to curries, stir-fries, soups and casseroles. Heating the turmeric in a little oil with black pepper will increase its digestive absorption.

Green tea
What for? Antioxidants
Great for active women due to its antioxidant activity, green tea reduces oxidative damage caused by intense exercise and environmental pollutants. It also contains a small amount of caffeine, stimulating mental function and energy, and making a good alternative to coffee and pre-workout supplements as it doesn't cause the crash often experienced after stronger stimulants. Green tea also possesses cancer preventative properties.
How do I take it?
Widely available, green tea is best steeped only for a few minutes as a bitter taste can develop if you brew it for too long.

Comfrey leaf
What for? Injuries
A traditional western herb, creams made from the leaves of comfrey plants can help to reduce pain and stimulate healing of injuries.
How do I use it?
Apply comfrey cream to sprains, strains and broken bones a few times per day until completely healed. Comfrey should not be ingested internally.

Ginger root
What for? Circulation
A fantastic herb for female surfers, ginger poooooooo circulation-boosting properties that help warm the body after a cold surf, and anti-inflammatory properties that help reduce muscle pain from intense workouts. Ginger also helps to reduce nausea and period pain.
How do I take it?
Ginger can be used fresh or dried in your daily cooking – grate fresh ginger onto salads and porridge or make a ginger, lemon and honey tea to warm you up on cool days.

Aloe vera
What for? Skin healing
The inner gel of the aloe vera leaf is soothing and cooling: Break open the leaves and squeeze the thick gel onto sunburnt skin, minor wounds or acne to cool the pain and assist healing. Studies show that the baby leaves possess more therapeutic value than the mature leaves, so pick the nice young fresh shoots.
How do I use it?
Use fresh aloe vera leaf gel or buy it in a bottle (but be sure to read the ingredients and make sure it has a considerable

amount of aloe vera in it). Apply the gel thickly onto the skin a few times per day for best effects.

....

Echinacea
What for? Immunity

High intensity training and getting cold in the surf can compromise immune function, leaving you susceptible to infections, but regular ingestion of Echinacea can support the immune system and prevent colds and flu. An especially good herb when travelling to third world countries, it can help your body fight off respiratory or gastrointestinal infections (such as diarrhoea) and support the healing of open wounds like reef cuts and sea ulcers.

How do I use it?

Echinacea can be bought as loose tea, tablets or tinctures. If you use the tea you can make it more palatable by mixing it 50/50 with peppermint tea.

Passionflower
What for? Relaxation

Nurturing and relaxing, passionflower can be used if you're feeling a little 'on edge' or can help you get a good quality night's sleep. Good quality rest is essential to maintain vibrant energy levels and a happy mood, and the gentle but effective passionflower will help you chill out without knocking you out. As well as being used for mental tension, it can help letting go of physical tension.

How do I use it?

Best drunk in herbal tea, passionflower combines well with chamomile and lemon balm for a relaxing cuppa. To assist with sleep drink a strong cup an hour before bed.

....

Flaxseed/ Linseed
What for? Long-term health

Flaxseeds are considered a 'functional food' with a wide range of health benefits including supporting healthy digestion and

contributing to overall anti-inflammatory omega 3 intake. Women transitioning into menopause can use flaxseeds to help balance the effect of fluctuating hormones. Recent studies also show flaxseeds may reduce the risk of breast cancer and support healthy blood pressure.

How do I take it?

You can buy whole or ground flaxseed, but it's preferable to buy it whole and grind it yourself in a blender, as the omega 3 oils are easily destroyed over time when the flax is pre-ground.

You can store freshly-ground flax meal in the fridge for a couple of weeks and add it to smoothies, baking, muesli, energy balls and pancakes.

The above herbal information is based on scientific studies and traditional herbal knowledge; it is not medical advice. If you suffer from allergies, health conditions, or are breast-feeding or pregnant, seek professional advice before using any herbs.

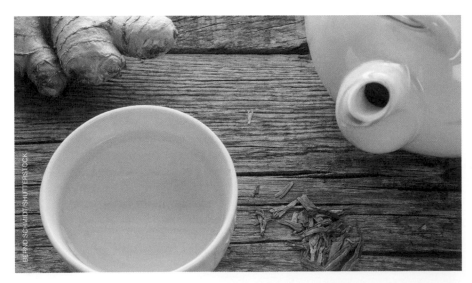

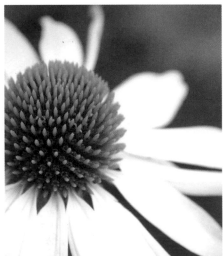

BERND SCHMIDT/SHUTTERSTOCK

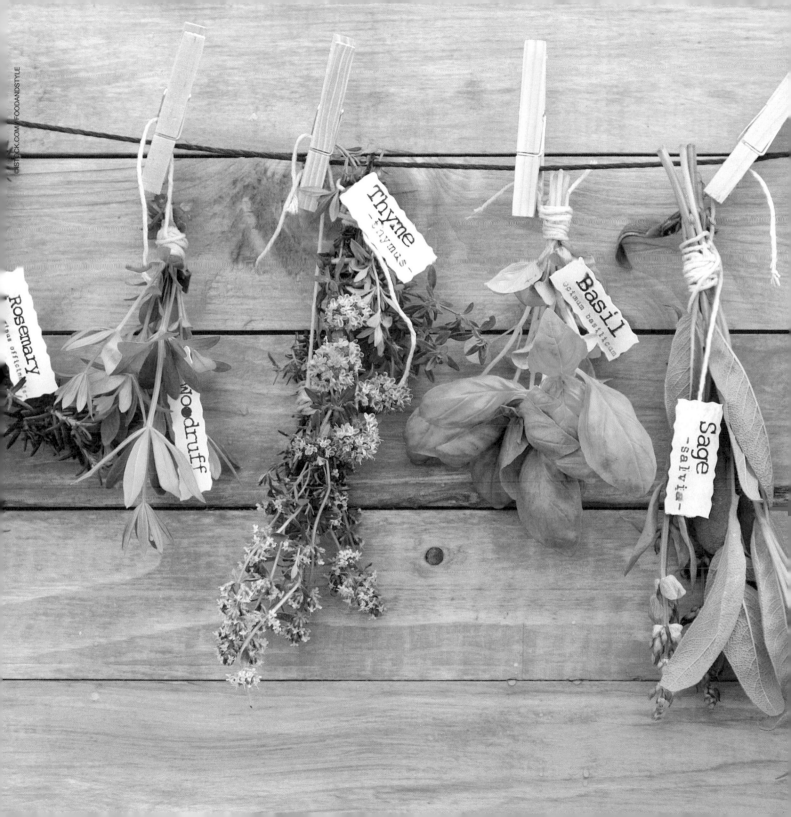

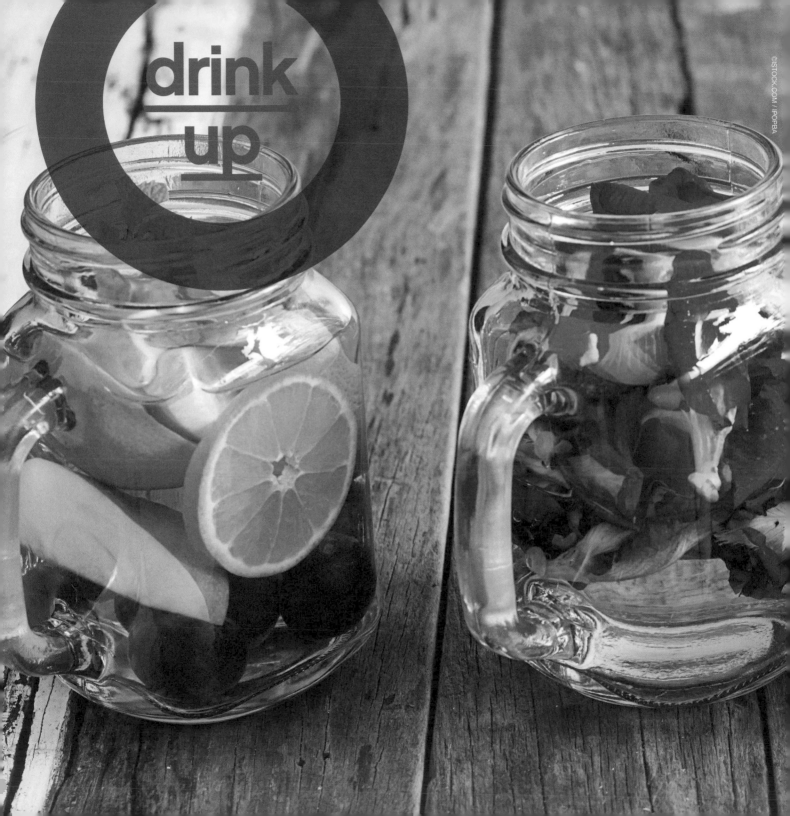

drink
up

Water intake is key to energy and vitality, and the importance of staying hydrated throughout the day, and especially during exercise, cannot be stressed enough.

Surfers are at particular risk of dehydration as you can be exposed to the sun for hours with no immediate access to drinking water, and despite being submerged in water you are still susceptible to sweating. It's vital to build hydration levels pre and post surf, as surfing without being well hydrated will decrease your energy levels, increase muscle cramps and lead to poorer surfing performance.

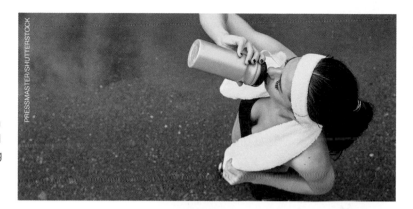

How much water do I need?

Women are made up of around 55% water, and over 14 years of age they require an average of 2 litres of water per day. This can include drinking water, other beverages such as milk and juice, and moisture in foods like fruit, vegetables and soup. Alcoholic beverages don't count as they have a dehydrating effect and caffeinated beverages are also thought to have a diuretic effect and shouldn't be counted as fluid intake.

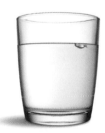

What does water do in the body?

• Assists with breakdown and absorption of nutrients in digestion
• Lubricates body tissues including joints, the gastrointestinal tract, the respiratory tract and eyes
• Maintains healthy skin, hair and nails
• Maintains body temperature
• Assists detoxification
• Keeps blood pressure and heart rate regular
• Supports healthy kidney function

Signs of dehydration

• Thirst*
• Dark coloured urine (anything darker than pale yellow)
• Fatigue
• Dry lips
• Dry skin
• Constipation
• Low mood
• Headache

* Don't rely solely on thirst as a sign of dehydration. You should also monitor how you are feeling, your urine colour and notice how your mouth and lips feel.

Test your skin hydration levels by pinching the back of the hand. The skin should naturally bounce back to place very quickly, if not you may be dehydrated.

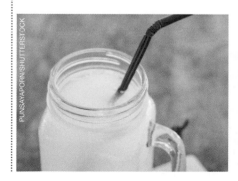

Tips to increase water intake

• Carry a drink bottle with you and sip from it throughout the day.
• Have a good drink of water before and after surfing.
• Add flavours to water using fruit: Squeeze the juice of ½ a lemon or lime into water or add berries, melon, peach, or herbs like mint, lemon balm or rosehip to give water a more pleasant taste.
• Fruit juice counts as fluid intake but is very high in sugar, so limit it to one small glass per day and try diluting it with water.
• Freshly squeezed vegetable juices can contribute to water intake. Great veggies for juicing include carrots, beetroots, celery, ginger, capsicum, cucumber and green leafy veggies such as baby spinach, wheatgrass and kale. Juices will also provide valuable electrolytes.
• Coconut water is very hydrating as it's a good source of water and potassium.
• Drink herbal tea. Popular flavours include peppermint, lemongrass, ginger, lemon, chamomile, liquorice, lavender, fennel and rosehip. Try turning them into ice teas for a cooling alternative.

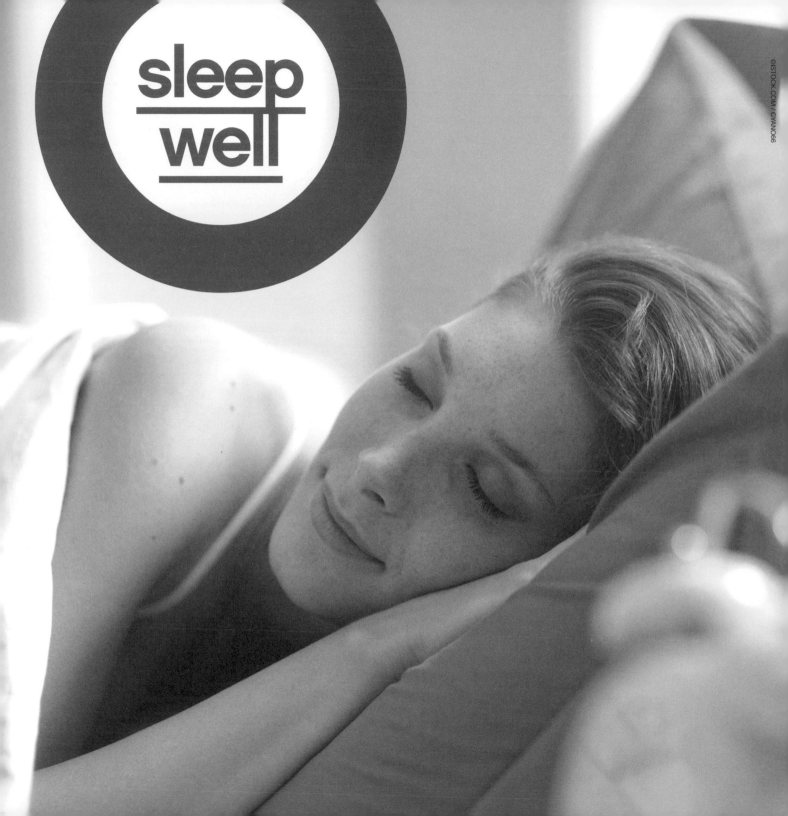

sleep
well

Why is sleep SO important?

Essential for maintaining your health, sleep is the body's natural cycle of self-restoration. While you're off in the land of nod, your body is busy repairing, detoxifying, rejuvenating and re-balancing.

Surfers need sleep to repair muscles and tissues, integrate new knowledge and re-energise. Most adults need around 8 hours of sleep per night, and studies show that having less than 6 hours can cause physical and psychological health problems.

What are the benefits of a good night's sleep?
- Reduced risk of injury during sport
- Improved concentration and memory
- Balanced immune function
- Reduced stress levels
- Healthier skin
- Healthy, natural detoxification
- Balanced metabolism and weight management
- Good energy levels
- Feeling happier and more relaxed
- Healthy heart and blood pressure

Sleep Well: Tips for a good night's sleep
Start a sleep routine
- Dim the lights in the evening to stimulate melatonin production – the body's natural sleep chemical.
- Switch yourself off from all mentally and visually stimulating activities 30 minutes before bed to allow the body to wind down. These include TV, study, computers, electronic tablets and mobile phones.
- Repeat the same pre-sleep routine each night – such as brushing your teeth, light reading and falling asleep on the same side of the bed.
- Go to bed and wake up at the same time each day. Going to bed earlier than midnight and waking early can improve the quality of your sleep. The age-old saying, 'one hour's sleep before midnight is worth two hour's sleep after midnight,' is true.

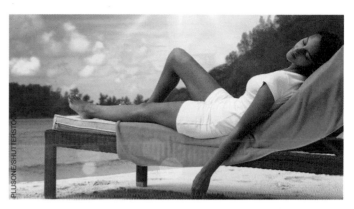

PLUSONE/SHUTTERSTOCK

Maintain a healthy routine by day
- Daily sunlight exposure of 30-60 minutes can improve sleep. When we're exposed to daylight our brain produces serotonin (the brain's natural happy chemical), and as the sun goes down and our eyes register darkness, this serotonin is converted to melatonin – a natural chemical that makes us fall asleep.
- Regular morning exercise can assist healthy bio-rhythms. Be aware that vigorous exercise in the evening can interfere with the body's natural sleep cycle.

Create a sleep-friendly bedroom
- Ensure your bedroom is dark and free from distracting lights and noises of TVs, computers and mobile phones.
- Ensure you have a comfortable pillow and mattress.
- Make sure there is good airflow and it's not too hot, as sleep requires our core body temperature to drop slightly.

Avoid sleep 'destroyers'
These include:
- **Caffeine** – a stimulant associated with sleep disorders and insomnia.
- **Alcohol** – this may help you get to sleep but it actually reduces the quality of your sleep and increases the chances of waking after a few hours.
- **Nicotine** – a stimulant that causes lighter sleep and can encourage you wake too early due to nicotine withdrawal.
- **Large meals at night** – going to bed on a full stomach can make it take longer to fall asleep.
- **Checking Facebook and electronic media in bed** – this increases sleep difficulty and can cause your mood to fluctuate during the day.

A VARIED AND WELL-BALANCED DIET SHOULD PROVIDE YOU WITH ALL THE ESSENTIAL INGREDIENTS NEEDED TO MAKE

ENERGY FOR SURFING

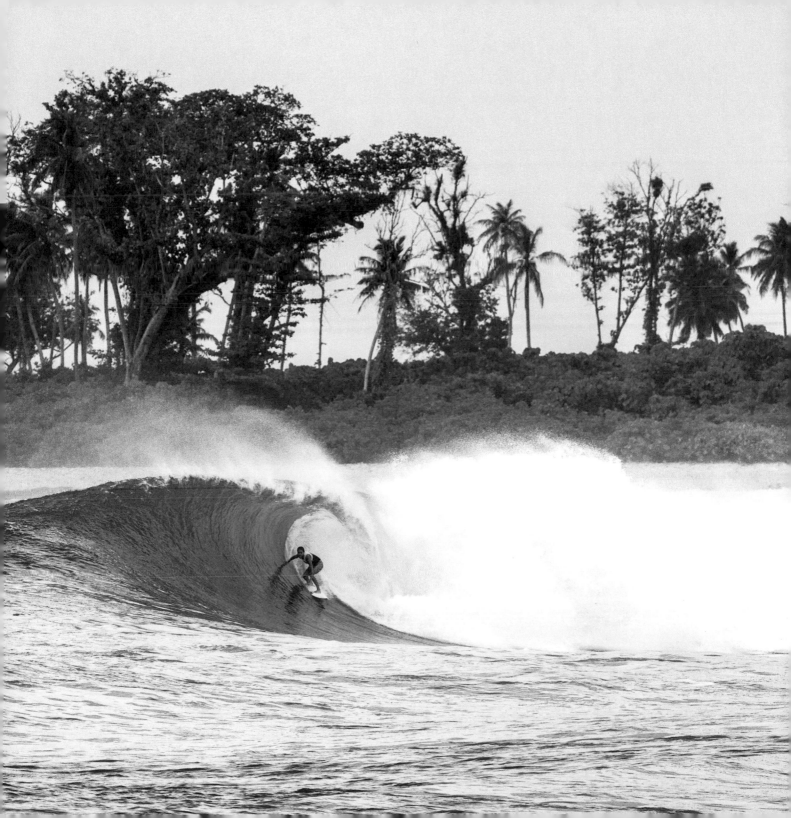

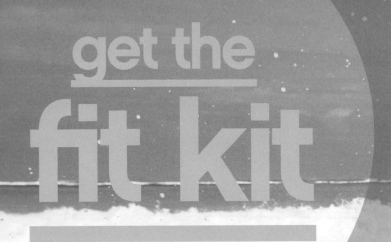

get the fit kit

Working out has never looked so good

These days there's a wealth of technical, stylish fitness wear for women. Using technical materials that are breathable, fast drying, odour resistant, anti-pilling, crease resistant and extra stretchy, the new fitness outfits are perfect for yoga, running, stretching and jumping. So we asked Roxy what they recommended from their fitness range, whatever you're doing celebrate getting sweaty in style!

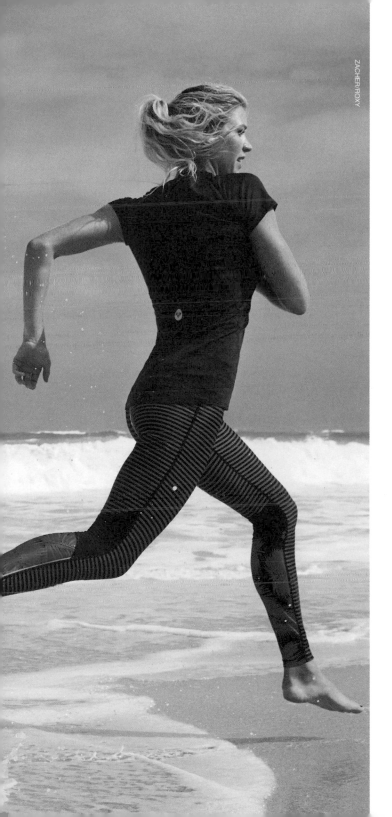

Best for Running

Roxy's latest collection has some key pieces for any running kit wardrobe. Pieces include new soft flatlock seamed leggings with an overlaid pair of mini shorts for extra coverage on cold days. Other pieces include cross back adjustable sports bra for extra support, running jacket with windproof material on the torso and light weight running windproof jackets.

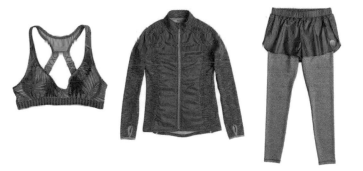

Best for Yoga

Yoga goddesses will love the Roxy yoga range. Key pieces include seamless leggings made from super stretch elastane and advance wicking technology. Eliminating chaffing and rubbing completely. Other products include large waist band leggings for even more comfort with quick drying fabric and a smooth cotton like feel. Complete the outfit with a fully lined sports bra with moisturising wicking jacquard fabric.

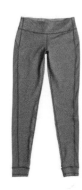
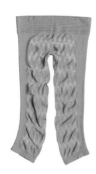
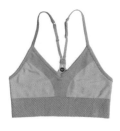

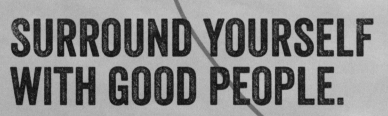

SURROUND YOURSELF WITH GOOD PEOPLE.

SUPPORTIVE PEOPLE CAN HELP YOU HEAD IN THE RIGHT DIRECTION WHEN YOU HIT A LOW POINT. A GOOD LAUGH WITH YOUR MATES WILL SOON PUT THINGS IN PERSPECTIVE!

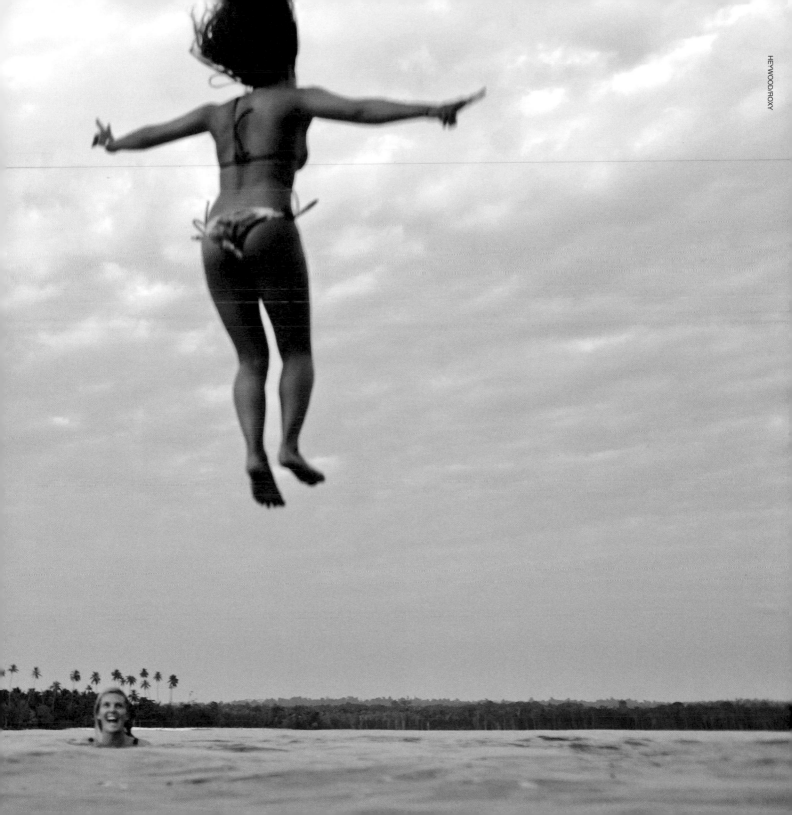

contributors

Meet our team of experts who contributed to this book.

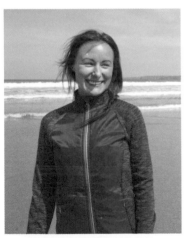

Aimee Stapleford

Aimee Stapleford is a Yoga Therapist based in Newquay, Cornwall. Aimee's passion for teaching yoga comes from the positive physical, mental and emotional changes that that she has seen within students.

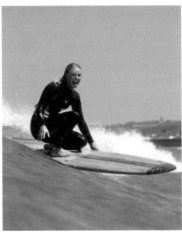

Nat Fox

Nat Fox is completely inspired by the sea. An ambassador for Roxy Fitness and Woodshed surfboards, Nat spends her time running the local ladies' surf club, teaching vinyasa, yin and SUP yoga plus running regular beach cleans for Surfers Against Sewage at home in Jersey.

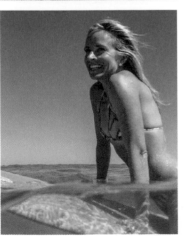

Hayley Shaw McGuinness

Hayley lives in Sydney and she is a fun, motivated and bubbly surf-a-holic. She understands the key to a happy life is healthy food, fitting in your daily workout and waking up with a smile. "Anything is possible in this life," says Hayley, "You just need to trust in your own heart that you can achieve what you set out to achieve."

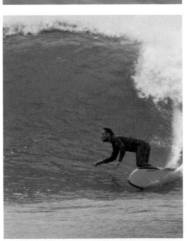

Lee Stanbury

Fitness instructor Lee Stanbury has 25 years experience in the fitness industry. He is an experienced head swim coach and personal trainer. He writes for various publications, invented the Powercord, is the MD of Big Blue Sports Distribution, fit4swimming.co.uk and fit2surf.com. In his spare time he finds time to pull into the occasional barrel at his local Cornish beach.

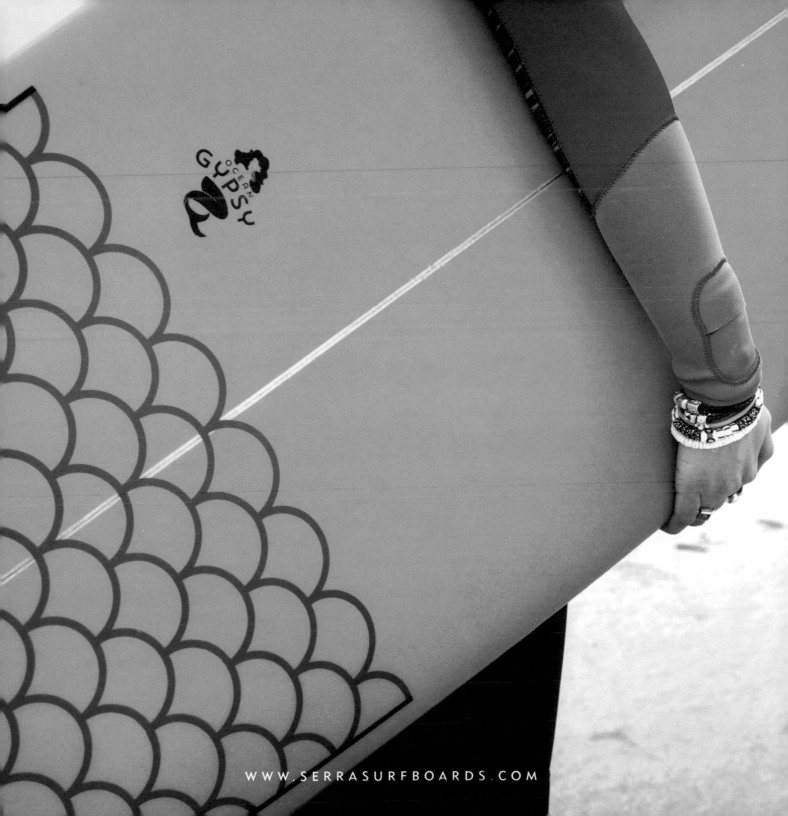

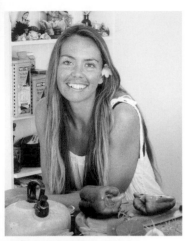

Samantha Bass

Samantha Bass is a qualified naturopath and specialist in holistic nutrition, herbal medicine and massage therapies in Australia. Sam's recipes are nutritional and fun... all natural using real, wholesome, functional foods. "Being a surfer myself I know the nutritional demands are high, and I know how much better I feel out in the surf after eating the right foods!" says Samantha.

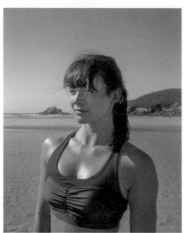

Jess Davis

Jess Davis owns the best café in Newquay: the Jam Jar, serving up healthy food and luscious gluten free cakes. In her spare time Jess also does a bit of modelling and since we asked her to do the fitness photos for us she has got hooked on boot camp!

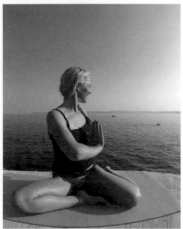

Katie Watson

Katie Watson is a Physio and Pilates Instructor, which gives her an amazing opportunity to share her passion for a healthy lifestyle. She loves to combine her job with making the most of the outdoors, so you will often find her teaching Pilates and yoga on paddle boards or at sunrise on the beach in her hometown of Torquay, Devon.

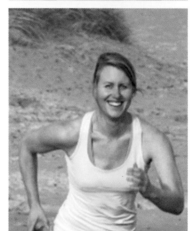

Nathalie Frankson

Nathalie specialises in teaching fitness at the beach or out in the countryside in Hampshire. Starting up her fitness company followmefitness.co.uk Nat explains, "I loved the energy and friends you meet through exercise so I knew I had to learn how to teach so that I could motivate and help others to feel energised themselves."

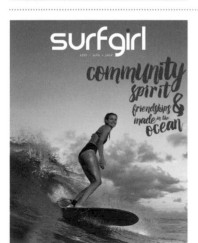

About SurfGirl

SurfGirl is the biggest global women's surfing magazine in print and online. SurfGirl magazine focuses on surfing, beach lifestyle, culture, fashion, fitness, health and wellbeing. SurfGirl is aimed at women who love surfing and surf culture.
www.surfgirlmag.com

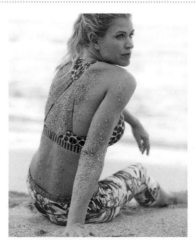

About Roxy

Roxy was born with a focus on surfing and carved her way to the mountains. Now Roxy Fitness focuses on yoga and running, offering the latest technology with the Roxy vibe and feel but never straying too far from the mountains and waves.
www.roxy.com

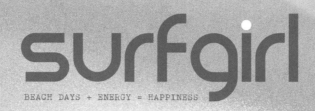

surfgirl

BEACH DAYS + ENERGY = HAPPINESS

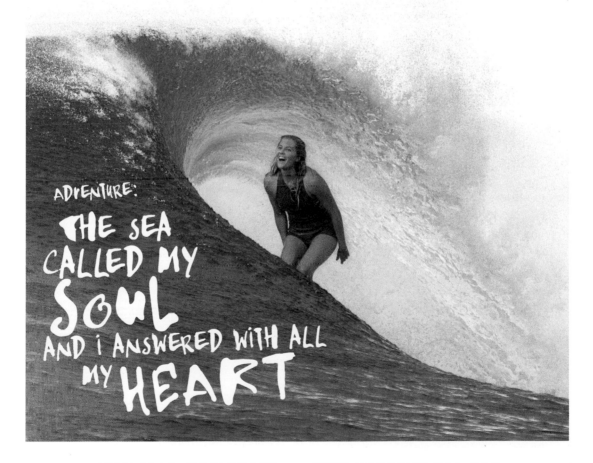

ADVENTURE:
THE SEA
CALLED MY
SOUL
AND I ANSWERED WITH ALL
MY HEART

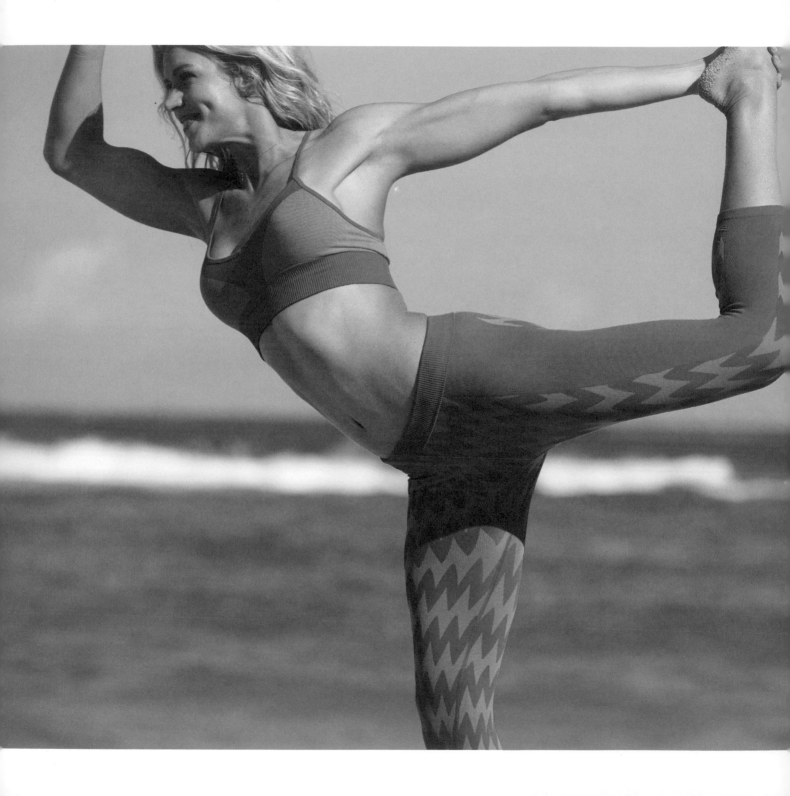

meet ROSY HODGE

South African surfer Rosy Hodge is a familiar face on the World Surf League world tour. Having hung up her contest rash vest a couple of years ago, she is now queen of the post-heat interview at WSL contests with her bubbly personality and winning smile.

Rosy, how does fitness improve your surfing?
The main way being fit benefits your surfing is by giving you confidence. The ocean is beautiful and it is also different everyday – some days you need to rely on your fitness to enjoy the challenges of being in the sea.

How many times a week do you train?
I love to run at least 3 times a week. When I am in a solid routine I'll run about 5 miles up to 5 times a week. I also try to go to Bikram yoga classes 3 times a week.

What areas do you focus on mostly, and why?
I find running is a good form of cardio and for me it is meditative, so it gives me time to think about surfing or whatever else is going on. I like Bikram yoga because I feel like the heat helps me to become more flexible. I take after my dad and we are both tall and inflexible, so I try work on my tight hips, hamstrings and lower back.

How do you stay positive and motivated?
It can be tricky; I'm on the road a lot, so I don't always get to my yoga class, but I can always put on my running shoes on and explore the area. I love the feeling after you workout – you are always happy you made the effort.

How important is it to eat healthily, and what does your typical daily diet entail?
Diet is so important: I wish I could put into practice what I know is good for me. I feel like I would be a happier human if I could stop eating so much sugar and junk food.

What would you tell someone learning to surf about how fitness is going to make it easier for them?
You'll enjoy surfing a lot more if you have some base fitness and understanding of your body. If you build muscle memory from working out, you can incorporate that into picking up surfing a lot more quickly.

What positive mantra sums up your life?
Action always beats intention.

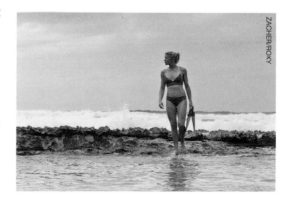

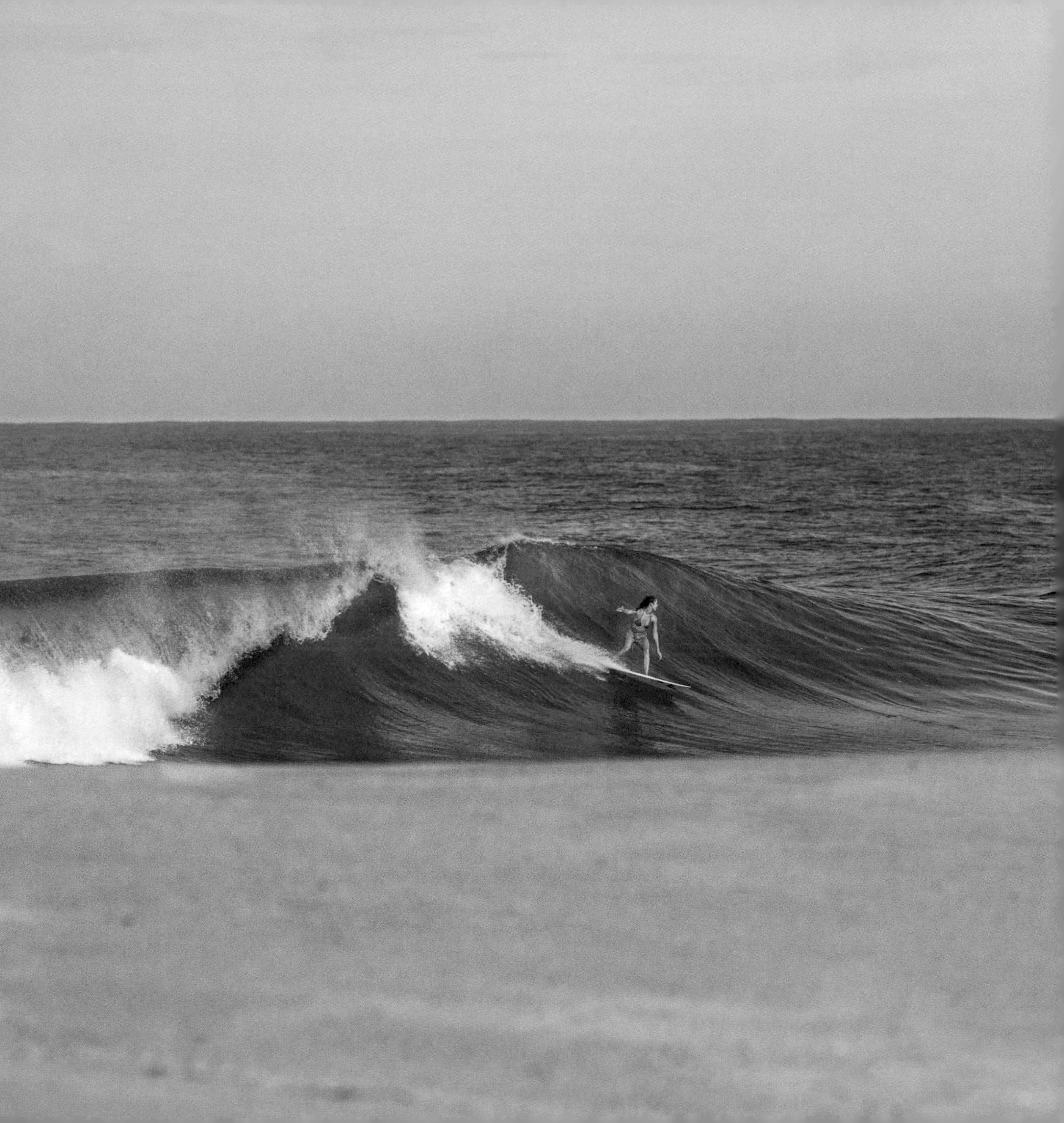
HEYWOOD/ROXY

meet MONYCA ELEOGRAM

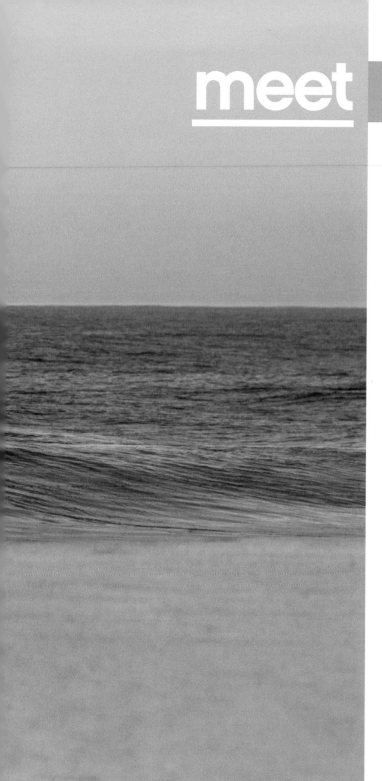

When free-spirited Roxy surfer Monyca Eleogram isn't at home in Maui, she's travelling all over the world, surfing and sharing her lust for life.

Monyca, how does fitness help your surfing?
Fitness is important for building endurance and will make you last longer in the water. It also helps prevent injuries. Core strength is also super-important in surfing because that is where the power in your surfing comes from.

How many times a week do you train?
Three or four, and I focus mostly on my core.

How do you stay positive and motivated?
I have so much to be happy about in my life. I live in a beautiful place and I have my husband Ola, who is wonderful. Both make me want to work hard so I can keep living this life in Maui that I am so grateful for.

What's on your workout playlist?
I mostly listen to dance music when I workout because it makes you want to move!

What does your typical daily diet entail?
I try my best to eat local, fresh and organic, and I stay away from junk food.

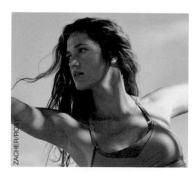
ZACHER/ROXY

What other sports do you do apart from surfing?
I love to play tennis and basketball.

What positive mantra sums up your life?
Live in love.

index

further reading

Available from surfgirlbeachboutique.com

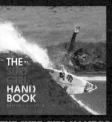

THE SURF GIRL HANDBOOK
By Louise Searle
ISBN 978-0-9523646-1-0

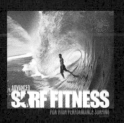

**ADVANCED SURF
FITNESS**
By Lee Stanbury
ISBN 978-0-9567893-9-6

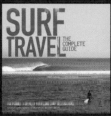

**THE COMPLETE GUIDE
TO SURF FITNESS**
By Lee Stanbury
ISBN 978-0-9523646-6-5

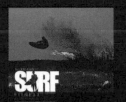

**SURF TRAVEL –
THE COMPLETE GUIDE**
Edited by Chris Power
ISBN 978-0-9523646-9-6

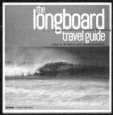

**THE LONGBOARD
TRAVEL GUIDE**
By Sam Bleakley
ISBN 978-0-9567893-4-1

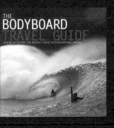

**THE BODYBOARD TRAVEL
GUIDE**
By Owen Pye with Rob
Barber and Mike Searle
ISBN 978-0-9567893-0-3

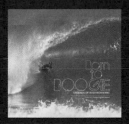

**BORN TO BOOGIE –
LEGENDS OF
BODYBOARDING**
by Owen Pye
ISBN 978-0-9567893-2-7

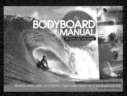

**THE BODYBOARD
MANUAL**
Edited by Rob Barber
ISBN 978-0-9567893-5-8

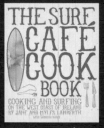

**THE SURF CAFÉ
COOKBOOK**
By Jane and Myles Lamberth
with Shannon Denny
ISBN 978-0-9567893-1-0

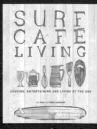

SURF CAFÉ LIVING
By Jane and Myles
Lamberth
ISBN 978-0-9567893-6-5

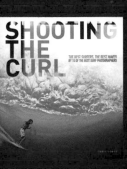

SHOOTING THE CURL
By Chris Power
ISBN 978-0-9523646-8-9

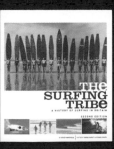

**THE SURFING TRIBE:
A HISTORY OF SURFING
IN BRITAIN**
By Roger Mansfield
ISBN 978-0-9523646-0-3

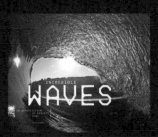

INCREDIBLE WAVES
By Chris Power
ISBN 978-0-9567893-3-4

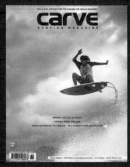

**CARVE SURFING
MAGAZINE**

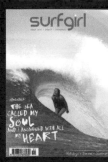

**SURFGIRL
MAGAZINE**

final tips

Whichever way you go with your training aim for regular sessions.

progression

Progression is key, exercises that mimic a surfing movement will always be best.

diversity

Diversify and change your programme subject to needs and requirements.

surf more

Always warm up, always cool down, surf longer, stay fitter and catch more waves!

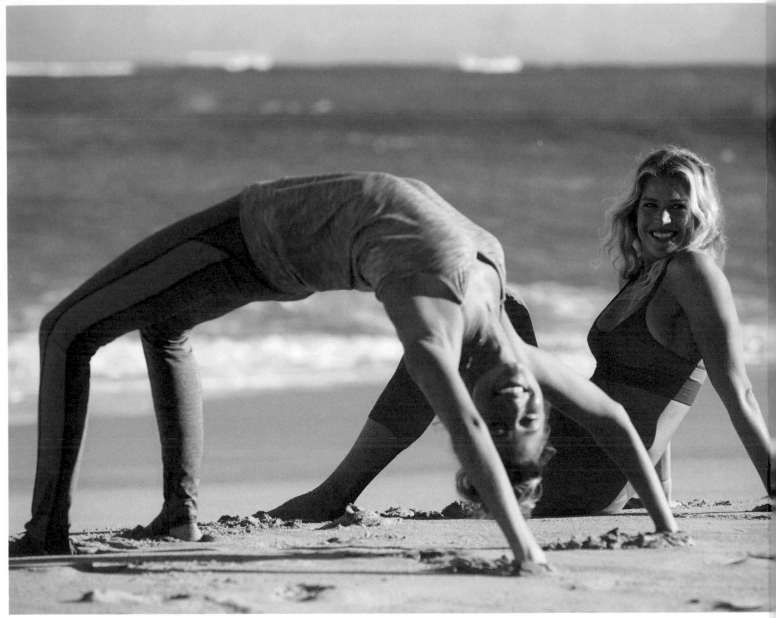

Monyca Eleogram & Rosy Hodge Professional Surfers | Paia, Maui | 20.913236° N, 156.401231° W | **#ROXYREADY**

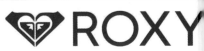 ROXY

Sun-Kissed
Sun-salutation